A GUIDE TO THE UNDERSTANDING OF ALZHEIMER'S DISEASE AND RELATED DISORDERS

A Guide to
the Understanding of

Alzheimer's
Disease
and Related Disorders

ANTHONY F. JORM

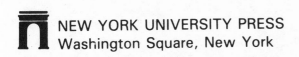

NEW YORK UNIVERSITY PRESS
Washington Square, New York

First published in paperback in the USA in 1989 by
New York University Press.
Washington Square.
New York, NY 10003

Library of Congress Cataloging-in-Publication Data

Jorm, A.F. 1951–
    A guide to the understanding of Alzheimer's disease
and related disorders.
    Bibliography: p.
    Includes indexes.
    1. Alzheimer's disease. 2. Dementia. I. Title.
    [DNLM: 1. Alzheimer's Disease. 2. Dementia.
WM 220 J82g]
    RC523.J67   1987   618.97'683   87-7929
    ISBN 0-8147-4170-3
            0-8147-4174-6 pbk

p 10 9 8 7 6 5 4 3 2 1
c 10 9 8 7 6 5 4 3 2

New York University Press books are printed on acid-
free paper, and their binding materials are chosen for
strength and durability.

Contents

Preface and Acknowledgements

An explosion of knowledge on the subject of dementia is currently occurring. This knowledge is hard to access except by reading technical journals across a range of disciplines. For researchers it is difficult enough to keep abreast of developments, but for practitioners it can be virtually impossible. The aim in writing this book is to communicate the rapidly expanding knowledge of dementia to practitioners and students in a form which is readily comprehensible to the non-specialist in the various disciplines concerned. The target audience includes medical practitioners, geriatric nurses, health administrators, social workers, clinical psychologists, occupational therapists and, perhaps occasionally, the interested lay person. This book is not intended as a guide to professional practice with demented people for any of these groups, but rather as a complement to existing expositions of professional practice with the elderly.

The organisation of the chapters is a little unconventional and deserves justification. It is tempting to discuss dementia starting with the microscopic aspects of the brain and working up to its social implications. However, I have preferred to begin by dealing with the social aspects of dementia before introducing more fundamental knowledge. The reason for this approach is basically motivational. By showing the enormous impact which dementia is going to have on the world in the near future, and how it may well affect our close relatives if not ourselves, I have hoped to motivate interest in the more fundamental scientific issues which follow. Inevitably, the book ends with the issue which interests people most — what can be done to manage dementia. Since the issue of management draws so heavily on fundamental knowledge of dementia, it is hard to place it anywhere but at the end.

This is the second book I have written. In the preface to the first (*The Psychology of Reading and Spelling Disabilities*), I admitted that I did not enjoy writing it. This time, however, I must say that I thoroughly enjoyed writing and found it very easy. Part of the change is due to greater experience of writing in the intervening years, but most of all it is due to the contrasting nature of the topics. Reading and spelling disabilities are a topic where there is little knowledge that is fully agreed upon. Consequently, there is little one can write without someone taking issue, and the realisation that this is the case makes writing difficult. With dementia, however, there is much agreement on fundamental matters and some firm foundations on which to build.

Many people have helped with this book. Particular thanks are due to those who read the earlier drafts and provided helpful comments which improved the final version immensely: Scott Henderson, Ailsa Korten, Peter Jorm, Louisa Jorm, Brian Hodge, Tim Hardwick, Yvonne Wells and an anonymous 'reviewer'. I cannot say I took all their suggestions, most notably the alternative title *Everything You Always Wanted to Know About Dementia but Have Forgotten to Ask*. Great help was also provided by Karen Maxwell and Penny Evans who typed several versions of the manuscript, and Jill Middleton who did the graphics work on the figures.

ACKNOWLEDGEMENTS

Table 1.1 is reproduced from Hughes, C.P. *et al.* A new clinical scale for the staging of dementia. *British Journal of Psychiatry*, *140*, 566–72, with permission of the author and publishers.

Figure 4.2 reprinted with permission of The Free Press, A Division of Macmillan Inc. from ALZHEIMER'S DISEASE: The Standard Reference edited by Barry Reisberg, M.D. Copyright © 1983 by Barry Reisberg, M.D.

Figures 4.3 and 4.4 are reproduced from *The Journal of Cell Biology*, 1985, 100, 1905–1912, by copyright permission of the Rockefeller University Press.

Figure 5.5 is reproduced from Moore, V. and Wyke, M.A. Drawing disability in patients with senile dementia, *Psychological Medicine*, Copyright Cambridge University Press, 1984.

Figure 6.4 is reproduced from Alter, M. Dermatoglyphic analysis as a diagnostic tool. *Medicine*, *46*, 35–56, © by Williams & Wilkins, 1967.

Table 10.1 is reproduced from Lipowski, Z.J. Transient cognitive disorders (delirium, acute confusional states) in the elderly. *American Journal of Psychiatry*, *140*, 1426–36, Copyright 1983, the American Psychiatric Association.

Table 11.1 is reproduced with the permission of M. Folstein.

Tables 11.9 and 11.10 are reproduced from Katz, S. *et al.* Studies of illness in the aged. The Index of ADL: A standardized measure of biological and psychosocial function. *Journal of the American Medical Association*, *185*, 914–19, Copyright 1963, American Medical Association.

Table 11.11 is reproduced from Kuriansky, J. and Gurland, B. The Performance Test of Activities of Daily Living. *International Journal of Aging and Human Development*, 7, 343–52, Copyright Baywood Publishing Company, 1976.
Table 11.2 is reproduced with the permission of A.S. Henderson.

1

What is Senile Dementia?

INTRODUCTION

Perhaps the simplest way to explain dementia is by way of an example. A typical instance comes from an article by Alois Alzheimer who was one of the pioneers in the study of dementia. Alzheimer (1907) described one of his cases in the following words:

> A woman, 51 years old, showed jealousy toward her husband as the first noticeable sign of the disease. Soon a rapidly increasing loss of memory could be noticed. She could not find her way around in her own apartment. She carried objects back and forth and hid them. At times she would begin shrieking loudly . . .
>
> Her ability to remember was severely disturbed. If one pointed to objects, she named most of them correctly, but immediately afterwards she would forget everything again. When reading, she went from one line into another, reading the letters or reading with a senseless emphasis. When writing, she repeated individual syllables several times, left out others, and quickly became stranded. When talking, she frequently used perplexing phrases and some paraphrastic expressions (milk-pourer instead of cup). Sometimes one noticed her getting stuck. Some questions she obviously did not comprehend. She seemed no longer to understand the use of some objects . . .
>
> The generalized dementia progressed however. After 4½ years of the disease, death occurred. At the end, the patient was completely stuporous; she lay in her bed with her legs drawn up under her, and in spite of all precautions she acquired decubitus ulcers.
>
> (from Wilkins and Brody, 1969, p. 110)

1

Alzheimer's description illustrates the important features of dementia. The woman had increasing problems with memory which progressed to the point where she could not remember even well-learned skills such as the way around her apartment. Eventually, all intellectual skills were lost. In addition, there were personality changes and socially inappropriate actions, including increased jealousy, a belief that someone wanted to kill her, and hiding objects in her apartment. As with most cases of dementia, it progressed until the victim's death.

All of these features are covered by more formal definitions of dementia. One of the more elegant and concise definitions comes from the Royal College of Physicians (1981):

> Dementia is the global impairment of higher cortical functions, including memory, the capacity to solve the problems of day-to-day living, the performance of learned perceptuo-motor skills, the correct use of social skills and control of emotional reactions, in the absence of gross clouding of consciousness. The condition is often irreversible and progressive (p.4).

There are two aspects of this definition which may be unfamiliar: *cortical functions* are the mental processes carried out by the cortex, or outer layer, of the brain, while *clouding of consciousness* refers to a lack of alertness in the person or lack of awareness of what is happening.

The American Psychiatric Association (1980) has proposed that the following features must be present for dementia to be diagnosed.

A. A loss of intellectual abilities which is severe enough to interfere with social or occupational functioning.

B. Memory impairment.

C. At least one of the following:

    (1) impairment of abstract thinking;

    (2) impaired judgement;

    (3) other disturbances of higher brain functions, involving language, complex sequences of action, perception, or construction;

    (4) personality change.

D. Not delirious or intoxicated.

E. Either of the following:

2

(1) evidence from the history, physical examination, or laboratory tests, of some organic factor which could plausibly produce the disorder;

(2) in the absence of such evidence, an organic factor can be presumed if other psychiatric disorders have been ruled out.

The aim of such diagnostic criteria is to be sufficiently specific so that different medical practitioners will diagnose dementia in a consistent manner. Perhaps the main weakness of these diagnostic criteria is that they do not tell us how much 'loss of intellectual abilities' or 'memory impairment' is required before dementia is diagnosed. In all cases of dementia the impairments are relatively slight at first, but can progress to the point where all skills of communication and self-care are lost, as with the case described by Alzheimer. The question then arises as to the point at which the affected individual is regarded as demented rather than normal. We obviously need some way of defining this point if consistent diagnoses are to be made from one practitioner to another. One solution is to regard dementia as a continuum of impairment. We could then label points on this continuum as *mild, moderate,* or *severe,* depending on the degree of dementia. However, it would still be important to ensure that descriptions such as *mild* or *severe* were used consistently by different people diagnosing dementia. Fortunately, useful methods for assessing the severity of dementia have been developed in recent years. One of these, the Clinical Dementia Rating, places people in one of five stages along a continuum from *health* to *severe dementia.* Within each stage of severity the typical features of the dementia are described in areas of memory, orientation, judgement and problem-solving, participation in community affairs, life at home and hobbies, and personal care. The overall scheme of this Clinical Dementia Rating is shown in Table 1.1.

DISORDERS PRODUCING DEMENTIA

Having now seen what dementia is, it is necessary to know what it is not. Although we speak of 'diagnosing dementia', it is not a disorder or disease in its own right. Dementia is, technically speaking, a *syndrome* or grouping of symptoms. There are many specific disorders or diseases which can give rise to this grouping of symptoms, all referred to as *dementia.* Although dementia is not a specific disorder, it is a very useful concept in practice, as are other

3

Table 1.1: Clinical dementia rating (CDR)

	Healthy CDR 0	Questionable dementia CDR 0.5	Mild dementia CDR 1	Moderate dementia CDR 2	Severe dementia CDR 3
Memory	No memory loss or slight inconstant forgetfulness	Mild consistent forgetfulness; partial recollection of events; 'benign' forgetfulness	Moderate memory loss, more marked for recent events; defect interferes with everyday activities	Severe memory loss; only highly learned material retained; new material rapidly lost	Severe memory loss; only fragments remain
Orientation	Fully oriented		Some difficulty with time relationships; oriented for place and person at examination but may have geographic disorientation	Usually disoriented in time, often to place	Orientation to person only
Judgement + problem-solving	Solves everyday problems well; judgement good in relation to past performance	Only doubtful impairment in solving problems, similarities, differences	Moderate difficulty in handling complex problems; social judgement usually maintained	Severely impaired in handling problems, similarities, differences; social judgement usually impaired	Unable to make judgements or solve problems

Community affairs	Independent function at usual level in job, shopping, business and financial affairs, volunteer and social groups	Only doubtful or mild impairment, if any, in these activities	Unable to function independently at these activities though may still be engaged in some; may still appear normal to casual inspection		No pretence of independent function outside home
Home + hobbies	Life at home, hobbies and intellectual interests well maintained	Life at home, hobbies and intellectual interests well maintained or only slightly impaired	Mild but definite impairment of function at home; more difficult chores abandoned; more complicated hobbies and interests abandoned	Only simple chores preserved; very restricted interests, poorly sustained	No significant function in home outside of own room
Personal care	Fully capable of self-care		Needs occasional prompting	Requires assistance in dressing, hygiene, keeping of personal effects	Requires much help with personal care; often incontinent

Source: Hughes et al. (1982)

syndromes like mental retardation and depression which similarly are not specific disorders.

Among the many disorders which can produce the syndrome of dementia are: Alzheimer's disease, multi-infarct dementia, Huntington's disease, Parkinson's disease, Pick's disease, depression and even AIDS. The obvious question is: why diagnose a non-specific syndrome of dementia rather than the specific disorders which give rise to it? The answer must be that, in practice, these disorders are often hard to tell apart. The concept of dementia can be regarded as a compromise diagnosis. In saying that someone is demented we are excluding a lot of other potential diagnoses which might explain mental impairment, such as mental retardation or amnesia (specific loss of memory). However, we are stopping at that point because it is difficult to diagnose any further. Amongst the elderly, whom we will define as people aged 65 or over, there are three main disorders which result in dementia. These are Alzheimer's disease, multi-infarct dementia, and mixed dementia resulting from a combination of the first two. It is these disorders which form the focus of Chapters 4 to 8.

Alzheimer's disease

Alzheimer's disease was first described by Alois Alzheimer using the case which was quoted earlier. After the woman's death, Alzheimer was able to examine her brain and noted changes which are regarded as characteristic of the disease which now bears his name. These changes are senile plaques and neurofibrillary tangles. The nature of these brain changes will be described more fully in Chapter 4. Until fairly recent times, Alzheimer's disease was regarded as a very rare disorder affecting people under the age of 65 only. Because it occurred in people who had not reached the conventional point of old age, it was described as a *presenile dementia*. At this time, dementias occurring in the elderly were labelled as *senile dementias*. These are much more common than the presenile Alzheimer's disease, and were generally thought to be due to cerebral atherosclerosis or narrowing of the arteries supplying blood to the brain. The brain was seen as being strangled of its blood supply because of diseased arteries, resulting in progressive dementia. However, autopsy studies on the brains of people with senile dementia, carried out in the 1960s and 1970s, showed that they in fact exhibited the characteristic features of Alzheimer's disease. It then became usual to refer to these people as suffering from *senile dementia of the Alzheimer type*. In more recent years, there has been a tendency to refer to all cases as *Alzheimer's disease*, irrespective of whether the disorder occurs before or after age 65. Thus, in the space of a few decades, Alzheimer's disease has been transformed from a rare dementia affecting those under 65 to one of the most common disorders affecting the elderly.

Multi-infarct dementia

The old concept of cerebral atherosclerosis was not completely off the mark. Although strangulation of the blood supply to the brain was not the cause of dementia, diseased arteries were later found to have a more indirect influence in producing dementia. Gradual narrowing of the arteries has been found to make people more prone to stroke because blockages of the blood supply occur more readily. A stroke, or *brain infarct*, results in death of the region of the brain to which the blood supply is blocked. After several strokes, sufficient brain tissue may be lost to result in dementia. This form of dementia, due to multiple strokes, was labelled as *multi-infarct dementia* by Hachinski, Lassen and Marshall in 1974, although the term *vascular dementia* is sometimes used to refer to the same disorder. Multi-infarct dementia is not as common as Alzheimer's disease in most parts of the world, but is still the second most common cause of dementia in the elderly.

Both Alzheimer's disease and multi-infarct dementia become more common with advancing age. It is not surprising, therefore, that elderly demented people are not infrequently found to suffer from a mixture of both disorders. This condition is often referred to as a *mixed dementia*, although it should not be regarded as a disorder in its own right.

Problems of diagnosis

These three common disorders causing dementia in the elderly are often difficult to tell apart. Although there are differences between the disorders which can allow a probable diagnosis in many cases, the only completely reliable way to diagnose them is by examination of the brain. The brain can be examined directly during life, but the risks of the surgical procedure involved are seldom justified for the

7

small benefits likely to be gained by the demented person. Therefore, certain diagnosis is presently only possible after death when the brain can be examined at autopsy. For this reason, the use of the global term *dementia* often becomes a useful description when the diagnosis of the specific disorders is difficult to make with certainty.

2

Impact of Senile Dementia on Society

PREVALENCE OF DEMENTIA

Although dementia can arise at any age, it becomes increasingly common after 65 years of age. In order to estimate the prevalence of dementia at various ages, it is necessary to survey people living in the general community, since only a minority of cases live in institutions such as nursing homes and many cases are not recognised by general practitioners. Many such community surveys have been attempted in the last few decades. Such a survey usually involves selecting a sample of elderly people at random from a list such as the electoral roll and then visiting them in their homes. After they have agreed to participate, a standard interview which assesses their mental functioning is carried out.

The results of three such surveys are shown in Table 2.1. These particular surveys have been selected because all deal with moderate and severe cases of dementia and they all indicate how common dementia is within quite specific age groups such as 65–69 years, 70–74 years etc. The most obvious finding in these surveys is that the prevalence of dementia rises steeply with age. Amongst those aged over 85, it is a very common problem indeed. It is also notable that there are differences between the surveys in the prevalence of dementia. For instance, dementia was found to be more prevalent in the English survey than in the Japanese one. However, such differences between the three surveys should not be taken too seriously, as they probably result from differences in the way the researchers defined a case of dementia.

9

Table 2.1: Surveys from three countries showing the percentage of the population suffering from moderate or severe dementia

Age group	England(%)	Japan(%)	New Zealand(%)
65–69	2.3	0.7	} 3.8
70–74	2.8	1.5	
75–79	5.5	2.2	6.4
80–84	} 22.0	7.7	11.0
85–89		} 17.7	23.6
90+			40.4

Sources: Kay *et al.* (1970), Karasawa, Kawashima and Kasahara (1982), Campbell *et al.* (1983)

AGEING OF THE POPULATION

Because dementia is most common in the very elderly, the prevalence of dementia in a society as a whole will depend on the proportion of its population that survives to be very old. For example, in a country where people rarely live to be over 65, dementia will not be a common problem, whereas in a country where a long lifespan is typical, it will be much more frequent. As inhabitants of the more developed countries of the world tend to have a longer lifespan than those of the less developed countries we would therefore expect dementia to be a greater problem in the more developed regions of the world. However, in all countries, both developed and developing, there is presently occurring a marked ageing of the population which will produce what has been called 'the coming epidemic of dementia' (Henderson, 1983).

It might be thought that this ageing of the population is due to the longer lifespans which people now enjoy. Although increases in lifespan do play a role, this factor is only of secondary importance. The major reason for the ageing of the population is a decrease in the number of children people are having. In the more developed countries there was a baby boom from the end of the Second World War until the mid-1960s. Since then these countries have had declining birth rates. The epidemic of dementia will reach a peak when the babies of these boom years become elderly from 2010 onwards. It is important to realise that the elderly people of this future time have already been born, so that future projections can be made with some certainty. Indeed, many of the readers of this book will be part of this future elderly boom.

Figure 2.1 show this ageing of the world in terms of the percentage of the population which is 60 and over. This graph is from the

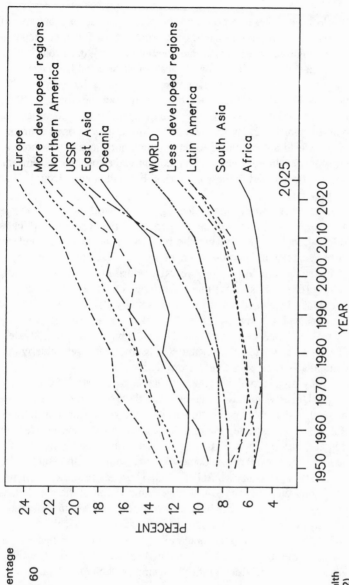

Figure 2.1: Percentage of the world's population aged 60 years and over: 1950–2025

Europe
More developed regions
Northern America
USSR
East Asia
Oceania
WORLD
Less developed regions
Latin America
South Asia
Africa

PERCENT

YEAR

1950 1960 1970 1980 1990 2000 2010 2020 2025

24 22 20 18 16 14 12 10 8 6 4

Source: World Health Organization (1982)

World Health Organization, and the points for future years are, of course, only projections based on current trends. It can be seen that the ageing phenomenon is already well under way in Europe, North America and the Soviet Union. Africa, South Asia and Latin America, on the other hand, are not even expected to reach by the year 2025 the position which the more developed countries had in 1950. However, this difference between the richer and poorer countries will only be shortlived. By the year 2075, the less developed countries of the world are predicted to have populations as aged as those of the more developed countries. Consequently, the epidemic of dementia will not be avoided in these countries, but will simply occur half-a-century later.

One other aspect of the ageing of the world's population is noteworthy. Not only will the porportion of the population which is elderly increase greatly, but the proportion which is very elderly (80+ years) will increase even more. To illustrate this point, in 1950 the very elderly (80+ years) comprised 13 per cent of the elderly (65+ years) in the more developed countries, and 8 per cent in the less developed countries. However, by 2075, the very elderly are expected to comprise 24 per cent of the elderly in the presently more developed countries and 21 per cent in the presently less developed countries. Significantly, it is among the very elderly that dementia is such an important problem.

Using population projections for the period 1980–2000 provided by the United Nations we can estimate the expected increase in the number of demented people in various countries of the world. Table 2.2 shows the expected increase for a number of countries over this 20-year period. These figures are based on the assumption that the age-specific prevalence of dementia is the same in all countries and that it stays the same over this period. Thus, the projected increases are purely due to changes in the age composition of the populations of these countries. As might be expected, the increase in the number of demented people will be greater in those countries which presently have relatively young populations. In the United Kingdom and Sweden, the increase will be smaller because these countries have already experienced a significant ageing of their populations.

INCREASED SURVIVAL OF THE DEMENTED

There is another important factor which will contribute to an increase in the prevalence of dementia in the future. This is the

Table 2.2: Expected increase in the demented populations of various countries, 1980–2000

Country	Projected increase(%)
Australia	52
Canada	51
New Zealand	44
United States	41
Sweden	16
United Kingdom	13

Source: Henderson and Jorm (1986)

increased survival of the demented elderly. In the past, many people suffering from senile dementia did not die from the disorder causing the dementia but from infectious diseases such as pneumonia. However, the discovery of various antibiotic drugs has led to the situation where pneumonia and other infectious diseases kill far fewer people who catch them than was the case earlier in the century. Although the control of pneumonia must be considered a major success in health care, it brought with it the consequence that people suffering from chronic incurable conditions such as dementia now live longer. Gruenberg (1977) has aptly referred to consequences of this sort as 'the failures of success'.

A number of pieces of evidence show that demented people are living longer than they used to. Gruenberg used information from a community survey of psychiatric problems carried out in southern Sweden in 1947 and again in 1957 to show that the demented elderly indentified in 1957 lived twice as long as those identified in 1947. Studies of demented patients admitted to hospitals have shown the same trend. For example, Christie (1982) found that 87 per cent of demented patients admitted to British hospitals in the 1940s were dead within 2 years, whereas in the 1970s only 55 per cent died during this period of time. Similarly, comparing the situation in the 1950s with that in the 1970s, Christie and Train (1984) found that only half as many demented elderly patients died within 12 months as had previously. The greatest increase in survival was for the very elderly demented patients aged 85 or over.

If the survival prospects of demented people continue to improve, there will necessarily be an increase in the percentage of the population who are demented at any particular time. This increase in the prevalence of dementia will occur even though the chance of someone becoming demented does not alter. In short, the 'success' of our ability to keep demented people alive longer may lead to the 'failure' of an

13

increase in the prevalence of dementia and add even further to the epidemic of dementia associated with an aged population.

THE ECONOMIC IMPACT

The young and old in a society must generally be supported by those of working age. As the population ages, the economic burden on the economically active section of the population will shift in its emphasis from supporting the young to supporting the old. Amongst the more developed countries there were 30.5 dependent elderly people for every 100 economically active people in 1960 and this will increase to 39 dependent elderly per 100 in the year 2000. However, this increased economic burden will be offset by a decrease in the number of dependent young from 90.3 per 100 economically active adults in 1960 to 74 in the year 2000. A similar pattern will occur in the less developed countries (Siegel and Hoover, 1982).

This shift in age of the economically inactive section of the population will have a major impact on the sorts of services a society needs to provide. Whereas children are to a large extent supported by their families, the elderly rely more heavily on the public purse. Furthermore, the public resources required by children are largely in the area of education, whereas those required by the elderly are more in the health and welfare areas. We can therefore expect public health expenditure to rise considerably, and senile dementia will make a large contribution to these costs, particularly as it often requires expensive hospital or nursing home care.

To give an example of the magnitude of the problem, one estimate puts the cost of caring for demented patients in the United States in the year 2030 as $30 000 000 000 in 1978-value dollars (Plum, 1979). This vast sum is eight times the amount now spent annually on *all* medical and mental health research in the United States; it makes current expenditure on research into dementia look miniscule. Given that the United States is a world leader in research on dementia, the expenditure of other advanced countries would look even more inadequate.

It hardly needs to be said that some way needs to be found to decrease the number of future cases of dementia. Although this may seem to be an ambitious goal there is every reason to expect it can be achieved. The majority of elderly people are not demented and, if we can discover the factors which differentiate them from those that are affected, we may have a basis for future preventive action.

3

Impact of Senile Dementia on Family Members

The problems of coping with a demented family member are already being faced by many people, but with the progressive ageing of the population few will remain untouched by the problems which dementia causes. Some of the problems are similar to those resulting from any serious chronic disease, but others are unique to dementia because no other impairment involves such a total destruction of the intellect and personality.

EARLY EFFECTS OF DEMENTIA ON FAMILY MEMBERS

Some idea of the early effects of dementia on family members comes from the problems discussed by participants of a support group for families of Alzheimer's disease patients (Barnes *et al.*, 1981). One of the first problems encountered is the stress involved with having the problem diagnosed. Early in dementia the changes are subtle and relatives will suffer uncertainty as to the nature of the problem. There may be years of frustration and worsening relationships. Even when dementia is diagnosed, the particular disease causing the dementia cannot be diagnosed with certainty in many cases. Once a diagnosis is made there is often an unmet need for information on what to expect in the future. Dementia can involve important personality changes such as irritability and restriction of activities which relatives can regard as spiteful or wilful on the part of the victim if they are not properly informed that such changes are due to a disorder of the brain. In order to lessen the emotional impact of a diagnosis of dementia, relatives may deny the problem by attributing it to a more minor disorder such as poor eyesight or hearing or they may believe that their loved one will be different from others

15

and get better. Once dementia has progressed to the stage where its effects are clearly evident, family members commonly feel a sense of loss as though the person they once knew were dead even though physically still present.

EFFECTS OF CARING FOR A DEMENTED RELATIVE

Most demented elderly people live in the community with relatives rather than in institutions. For this reason relatives often have the difficulties of caring for a severely disabled person in addition to the emotional distress of seeing a loved one become demented. Several attempts have been made to find out the aspects of the demented person's behaviour that family members find most difficult to cope with and to assess the ill-effects that these have on caregivers themselves.

Greene and his colleagues (1982) discovered two broad classes of behaviour disturbance that relatives find difficult to tolerate. The first is passive, withdrawn behaviour as seen in the demented person who sits around all day, has few interests, and does not interact with other family members. This behaviour pattern caused considerable personal distress in family members. They tended to feel that they could not cope, became depressed, and felt that their own health was suffering. The second class of behavioural disturbance causing problems to relatives was unstable mood. Demented people with this pattern became moody, angry and accusing. Relatives tended to react with negative feelings towards them; they felt embarrassed, angry and frustrated with the demented person. Surprisingly, there were other major problems in demented people which were generally well tolerated by relatives. The demented person's low level of mental functioning and their inability to perform everyday self-care skills did not so greatly upset relatives.

Other researchers have attempted to identify quite specific problems which relatives find difficult to bear. Argyle, Jestice and Brook (1985), for example, interviewed caregivers of elderly people admitted to a psychogeriatric unit of a hospital because they could no longer be coped with at home. Most of these elderly people suffered from senile dementia. The frequency of various problems reported by the caregivers is shown in Table 3.1. The most common problems in the elderly person were being unable to dress unaided, being restless by day, urinary incontinence, and causing sleep disturbance. The caregivers frequently reported embarrassment, anxiety

16

Table 3.1: Problems reported by relatives caring for a demented elderly person

	Percentage of relatives reporting the problem	Percentage of relatives not coping with or not tolerating the problem
Problems due to patient's behaviour or limitations		
Unable to dress unaided	69	9
Restless by day	52	41
Urinary incontinence	50	19
Inappropriate urination	24	60
Sleep disturbance	48	43
Help with washing	48	13
Communication impairment	44	41
Uncooperative	40	32
Falling	40	12
Faecal incontinence	37	34
Faecal smearing	23	57
Aggression	35	50
Wandering	30	50
Verbal abuse	27	59
Irresponsible/dangerous behaviour	27	18
Help with transfer to commode needed	27	6
Unable to walk unaided	24	7
Cannot walk at all	6	25
Deafness	21	15
Feeding difficulties	18	55
Poor vision	16	40
Other physical illness	13	25
Relatives' own limitations or problems		
Embarrassment	58	6
Anxiety/depression	51	6
Personality conflict	29	28
Weakness	27	24
Lack of confidence	20	8
Arthritis	16	20
Shortness of breath	15	11
Other illness	13	13
Social problems associated with patient's care		
Decreased social life	74	13
Cannot leave for 1 hour	45	13
Conflicting family demands	40	10
Stairs in the home	23	7
Too much washing (clothes)	18	18
Overcrowded home	13	0
Too far to shops	13	0
Financial burden	6	25

Source: adapted from Argyle, Jestice and Brook (1985)

or depression, and a decreased social life due to the elderly person's behaviour. However, many of these common problems could be coped with by the caregivers, while other less frequent problems caused great difficulties. The problems that caregivers could least cope with were inappropriate urination, smearing of faeces, aggression, wandering, verbal abuse, and feeding difficulties.

The common factor to most of these problems seems to be that they demand so much of the caregiver's time, a conclusion echoed by the comments of participants in the support group for relatives described by Barnes and colleagues (1981):

> A major problem mentioned by all group members was the great amount of time required to care for even a mildly impaired Alzheimer patient at home. As patients become progressively more demented, the spouse assumed almost total care for the patient and soon felt trapped by the time and effort required. One group member said that the demands of caring for his wife were so great that he was a 'prisoner of love'. The daughter of another patient said: 'My father does everything for my mother except breathe'. Spouses spent so much time looking after the patient that they seemed to identify themselves with the patient and often lost sight of their own personal needs and interests. When one patient was hospitalized for an acute episode, his spouse stayed with him at the hospital day and night. Later she realized that it would have been more reasonable to have taken a much needed vacation, but she had become so used to the idea that her husband could not get along without her that she stayed with him even in the hospital (p.82).

THE HIDDEN COSTS OF HOME CARE

With the future increase in the number of demented people, and the consequent increase in the demand on health services, it will not be surprising if governments attempt to reduce costs by encouraging care of the demented at home wherever possible. It has been demonstrated by Doobov (1980) that the cost of home care services such as home nursing, home helps, meals-on-wheels, pharmaceuticals, doctors' visits, paramedical services etc. is always cheaper than hospital care and is virtually always cheaper than nursing home care as well. Taking into account the full resource costs of home care by including the additional costs of accommodation, food, heating and fuel, home care still always costs less than hospital care (even for persons living alone). For patients who live with their families and receive unpaid assistance from them, home care is nearly always cheaper than nursing home care. From a purely economic point of view, therefore, home care looks like a desirable alternative. There are, however, other costs of home care which are ignored by the economist because they are difficult to value in money terms. These include the value of the assistance the caregiver provides and, perhaps more importantly, the cost in stress which caring for a demented person produces. These are the hidden costs of home care. Eventually the point may be reached where the personal cost to family members is so great that they can no longer look after the demented person and must seek institutional care. Indeed, the major reason for elderly demented people being admitted to a day hospital in Scotland was reported to be that the family was unable to cope with full-time care (Greene and Timbury, 1979).

The extent of the emotional cost to caregivers has been studied by Gilleard and his colleagues (1984). They assessed the extent of psychiatric disturbance in the caregivers of mentally infirm elderly people who were attending or about to attend day hospitals. Using a brief screening questionnaire Gilleard and his colleagues found well over half the caregiving relatives to be psychiatrically disturbed. Using the same questionnaire, other researchers have found, by contrast, that less than a quarter of the general community have a psychiatric disturbance. However, not all caregivers were found to be equally prone to psychiatric disturbance. Women caregivers, who make up the vast majority of relatives giving care to the demented elderly, appear to suffer more than men. Not surprisingly, greater disturbance in caregivers was found when the demented person showed more of the sort of problems listed in Table 3.1. It was also greater when the caregivers viewed their own health as being poorer and considered their past relationship with the elderly person was not good. Any measures to reduce the stress on caregivers would be of obvious benefit. Indeed, day hospital attendance by the elderly person did seem to reduce stress a little. Unfortunately, support received from other family members and professional help were not related to reduced stress on caregivers, perhaps indicating there is little the community can do to help in this regard. However, other research has shown that visits by other relatives to the demented person do relieve the caregiver's feeling of burden (Zarit, Reever and Bach-Peterson, 1980) and that home help and community nursing services boost morale and relieve distress (Gilhooly, 1984).

THE NEED FOR ACTION

It has been found that elderly demented people who are cared for by family members are less likely to become long-stay residents in institutions (Bergmann *et al.*, 1978). Family members who care for demented people are clearly doing the community a service by reducing the financial burden on the state and are possibly providing more satisfactory care for the demented at the same time. However, this service is provided at considerable personal cost. Alarmingly, Bergmann and his colleagues (1978) found that in Britain these families were not receiving the degree of social services they warrant. Rather, services tend to go to those living alone who are the least likely to be able to stay in the community anyway. There is a clear need for governments and the community to acknowledge the important service given by caregiving family members and to provide them with help and relief from stress.

4

Brain Changes in Alzheimer's Disease

In the first three chapters we have looked at dementia as a global syndrome. Now we will turn to specific disorders which can produce dementia. This chapter, and the three that follow it, look in detail at the most common cause of dementia in the elderly — Alzheimer's disease.

PLAQUES AND TANGLES

Alzheimer's disease cannot be diagnosed with certainty during life, but at autopsy it can be recognised by certain microscopic changes in the brain. Although many changes occur in the Alzheimer brain, the most important for establishing a diagnosis are *senile plaques* and *neurofibrillary tangles*. These changes were recognised early this century by Alois Alzheimer, after whom the disease was subsequently named.

To understand the nature of these changes it is necessary to know something about the structure of individual neurons, since it is at this level that the changes occur. For readers whose knowledge of neurophysiology may be rusty, Figure 4.1 shows an idealised diagram of a neuron which highlights the important features. The first features to note are the tree-like branches called *dendrites*. These receive chemical messages from other nerve cells. The messages are conducted to the *cell body* and then sent down the *axon* to be transmitted to the dendrites of other neurons. The messages from a single axon may be sent on to the dendrites of a great many other neurons.

Senile plaques occur in areas of the brain containing axons. A picture of one is shown in Figure 4.2. Senile plaques consist of a core of protein called *amyloid* which does not occur naturally in the

Figure 4.1: The important features of a nerve cell

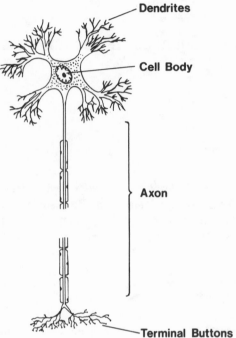

Dendrites

Cell Body

Axon

Terminal Buttons

Figure 4.2: A senile plaque

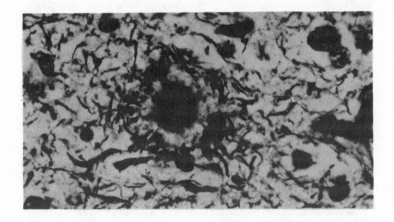

Source: Wisniewski (1983)

brain and is surrounded by debris from degenerating neurons. Plaques undoubtedly interfere with the messages being sent from one neuron to another. However, why they form is presently unknown.

Neurofibrillary tangles, on the other hand, occur in the cell body of brain neurons. They consist of bundles of long thread-like structures as shown in Figure 4.3. When examined closely, these threads are found to consist of filaments twisted around each other in pairs to make a helix. The twisting together of these filaments produces the scalloped appearance of the thread-like structures shown in Figure 4.4. As with plaques, nobody is sure why neurofibrillary tangles form. However, they may derive from normal structures in neurons called *neurofilaments*. These are long fibres which run parallel to the long axis of the neuron. Neurofilaments are believed to play a role in the transport of essential chemicals around the nerve cell, for example, from the cell body to a distant axon. One theory is that neurofibrillary tangles form when there is some interference with the transport function of the neurofilaments in a neuron (Gajdusek, 1985).

Plaques and tangles occur in normal elderly people as well as in those with Alzheimer's disease. However, they are much more frequent in Alzheimer's disease brains than in normal elderly brains. The majority of people in their late 50s and early 60s have been found to have some plaques and tangles (Ulrich, 1985). By the time people reach their 90s, few are totally without plaques and tangles, although still only a minority are severely affected. Table 4.1 shows the percentage of people dying at particular ages who have many plaques and tangles in their brains.

REGIONS OF THE BRAIN AFFECTED

Plaques and tangles do not occur equally in all parts of the brain. They tend to be more common in some regions than in others. The most prominently involved regions are the *hippocampus* and the *cerebral cortex*.

The location of the hippocampus can be seen in Figure 4.5, which shows a diagram of the brain. There are actually two hippocampi in the brain, one lying to the left side of the brain's interior and the other to the right side. The hippocampus is known to have a vital role in memory. People who have had both their hippocampi removed by surgical operation are virtually without the ability to

Figure 4.3: A fragment of a neurofibrillary tangle is shown in (b). The thread-like structures which make up the tangle can be seen. Portions of the tangle marked with arrowheads in (b) are shown at greater magnification in (a) and (c)

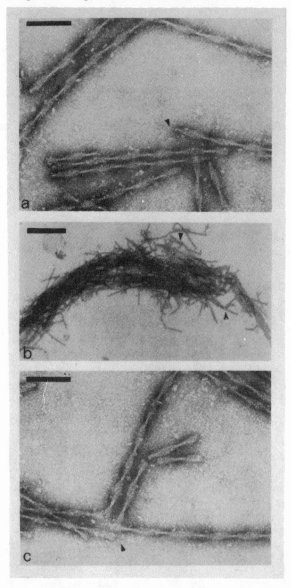

Source: Wishchik *et al.* (1985)

Figure 4.4: The twisted pairs of filaments which make up a neurofibrillary tangle. The scalloped edges are due to the twisting of the filaments

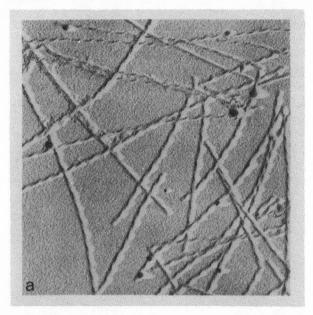

Source: Wischik *et al.* (1985)

Table 4.1: Percentage of people dying at different ages affected by many plaques and tangles

Age in years	Percentage affected
< 55	0
55–64	3
65–74	5
75–84	20
85 +	45

Source: adapted from D.F. Miller, *et al.* (1984)

learn new material, although their memory for the past before their operation is intact. For example, one such patient moved house after his operation, but was unable to recall his new address even a year afterwards. However, he still remembered his old address. He would also read the same magazines over and over because he could not remember having read them before (Milner, 1966). As we have

Figure 4.5: Cholinergic nerve cells from the basal forebrain (BF) send long axons up to areas of the cortex (C) and to the hippocampus (H)

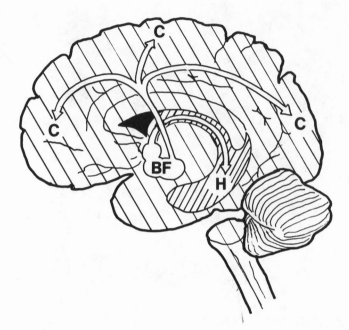

Source: adapted from Coyle, Price and DeLong (1983)

seen, dementia always involves problems of memory and in Alzheimer's disease these may be due to damage to the hippocampus. Indeed, it has been found that many of the nerve cells connecting the hippocampus to other areas of the brain are lost in Alzheimer's disease (Hyman *et al.* 1984) with the end result that it is unable to play its important role in memory. Some scientists have gone so far as to argue that damage to the hippocampus is the basic cause of most of the mental impairments seen in Alzheimer's disease because this is the region found most consistently to be involved in the disease (Ball *et al.*, 1985). Fortunately, however, the brains of Alzheimer's disease sufferers may be able to compensate to some extent for this progressive loss of neurons. It has recently been observed that the remaining hippocampal neurons sprout and form new connections with other neurons to replace those lost (Geddes

Figure 4.6: Diagram of a synapse, showing the terminal button of one neuron (left) and receptors of the other (right). The gap between the two is bridged by a chemical known as a neurotransmitter

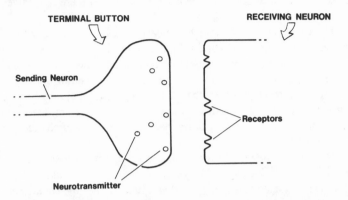

et al. 1985). This finding raises the exciting possibility that therapies could be developed to slow down the loss of function in Alzheimer's disease by facilitating the formation of new neural connections.

The other region of the brain severely affected by plaques and tangles is the cerebral cortex which is the surface layer of nerve cells covering the brain. The cerebral cortex is the centre for various complex mental processes such as initiating voluntary actions, language and speech, perceiving the world, and finding one's way around unfamiliar environments. In short, the cortex is vital to much of human intelligence. Involvement of various parts of the cortex is thought to explain certain mental impairments often (but not always) seen in Alzheimer's disease (Cummings and Benson, 1983). Damage to the cortex can produce problems with language, performance of actions on command, and recognition of familiar objects. These impairments will be discussed in greater detail in the next chapter.

NEUROTRANSMITTERS IN ALZHEIMER'S DISEASE

When messages pass from the axon of one neuron to the dendrites of others, they must pass over a small gap separating the two. The point at which messages pass is known as a *synapse* and is shown in Figure 4.6. The diagram represents a considerable magnification of the structures shown at the tips of the neuron in Figure 4.1. The gap at the synapse is bridged when the neuron sending the message releases a chemical known as a *neurotransmitter* from its terminal buttons. The neuron on the other side of the gap has receptors for detecting the presence of the neurotransmitter and thereby receives the message.

There are many different chemicals believed to act as neurotransmitters in the human brain. In fact, neurons are often described in terms of the particular type of neurotransmitter they use. Because of the important role neurotransmitters play in sending messages from one neuron to another, there has been much interest in finding out whether Alzheimer's disease involves deficiencies in particular neurotransmitters. Such specific neurotransmitter deficiences do indeed occur.

The strongest evidence for such a deficiency involves the neurotransmitter *acetylcholine*. The system of neurons which uses acetylcholine as its neurotransmitter is often referred to as the *cholinergic system*. As with plaques and tangles, neurotransmitters can only be directly studied after death. However, here there is an even greater complication in that chemical changes rapidly occur once the brain is dead, so that neurotransmitters can only be studied very soon after death. For this reason, acetylcholine itself is seldom studied. Instead, an enzyme called choline acetyltransferase (CAT for short) is used as an indicator of the neurotransmitter because it remains relatively stable in the brain for hours after death. CAT is used by the neurons to manufacture acetylcholine, so any severe lack of it would affect levels of the neurotransmitter itself. Several studies have shown that CAT levels are markedly reduced in Alzheimer's disease, and the degree of reduction is strongly related to the severity of the dementia before death (Perry *et al.*, 1978).

Many of the cholinergic neurons which send messages to the cortex actually have their cell bodies lower down in the *basal forebrain*, particularly in an area of the basal forebrain known imposingly as the *nucleus basalis of Meynert*. These neurons send long axons up to the cortex and to the hippocampus as shown in Figure 4.5. It has been found that many of the cholinergic cells originating from the basal forebrain have died in the brains of Alzheimer's patients (Coyle, Price and DeLong, 1983). The loss of cholinergic neurons in the basal forebrain has been explained in two ways. One theory is that Alzheimer's disease occurs when the nerve cells in the basal forebrain degenerate for some reason. Because the basal forebrain sends axons up to the cortex and hippocampus, loss of neurons from this small region of the brain could result in a widespread loss of CAT. However, this theory is disputed by others who see the hippocampal and cortical abnormalities as the primary problem and regard the loss of neurons from the basal forebrain as being a consequence of these. Whatever the causal direction, loss of cholinergic neurons appears to be an important factor in Alzheimer's disease. Evidence from monkey brains indicates that degenerating cholinergic neurons may also be a source of senile plaques, one of the characteristic features used in diagnosing Alzheimer's disease *post mortem* (Struble *et al.*, 1982).

To add further weight to the importance of the cholinergic system in Alzheimer's disease there is evidence that normal adults show mental impairments similar to those in mild Alzheimer's disease when given drugs which disrupt acetylcholine. One such drug, *scopolamine*, acts by blocking receptors (shown diagrammatically on the receiving neuron in Figure 4.6) so that they are insensitive to acetylcholine. In one study where scopolamine was given to normal adults (Drachman and Leavitt, 1974), they became worse at storing new information in memory, at finding information already stored in memory, and at intelligence tests involving unfamiliar problems. In some cases, scopolamine produces severe deficits which are quite like those in dementia. Serby and his colleagues (1984) described a 40-year-old man who experienced major changes for at least 10 hours after receiving scopolamine in an experiment. He had difficulty speaking, his memory for recent events was severely impaired, he experienced visual illusions, had difficulty finding his way around, was confused, and showed impaired judgement.

Although deficiencies of the cholinergic system appear to play an important role in producing the mental impairments of Alzheimer's disease, other neurotransmitters are likely to be involved as well. One such neurotransmitter is *somatostatin* which is used by certain neurons in the cerebral cortex. Not only are levels of somatostatin greatly reduced in Alzheimer's disease (Beal *et al.*, 1985), but neurons using this neurotransmitter appear to be affected by plaques and tangles (Morrison *et al.*, 1985; Roberts, Crow and Polak, 1985). More recently, levels of a third neurotransmitter, *corticotropin-releasing factor*, have been found to be greatly reduced in the cortex (De Souza *et al.*, 1986). However, the role that these neurotransmitters might play in producing the mental impairments of Alzheimer's disease is still not known.

USE OF BRAIN IMAGING TECHNIQUES IN ALZHEIMER'S DISEASE

The study of brain changes in Alzheimer's disease is greatly limited by the fact that the human brain is generally accessible for direct examination only after death. However, to understand brain changes in Alzheimer's disease fully it is necessary to observe the progression which occurs from normal functioning to severe dementia. Brain imaging techniques, which give information about the brain during life, may provide at least a partial solution to this problem. There are three major techniques of brain imaging in current use: computerised axial tomography (CT), magnetic resonance imaging (MRI) and positron emission tomography (PET). CT scans have been in use for over a decade, while MRI and PET are both fairly new.

CT scanning is an X-ray technique in which the attenuation of the X-rays by different parts of the brain is analysed by computer to produce an image. The resulting image shows differences in tissue density between various brain regions. In routine use, CT scans are inspected visually to locate any gross brain changes. The gross changes occurring in Alzheimer's disease are atrophy (shrinkage) of the brain and enlargement of the ventricles (cavities in the brain containing cerebrospinal fluid). Unfortunately, atrophy and ventricular enlargement are not specific to Alzheimer's disease. Rather, they occur as part of the ageing process, although there is some evidence that atrophy is greater in Alzheimer's disease than in normal ageing (McGeer, 1986). A more promising approach has been to study differences in tissue density in a quantitative manner, rather than use visual inspection of the CT image. As well as a visual image of the brain, the CT scanner can produce density numbers, each of which reflects the density of tissue in a quite small region of the brain. Although there are numerous technical problems involved with this approach, there has been a general finding of reduced brain tissue density in Alzheimer's disease (Albert *et al.*, 1984; Bondareff, Baldy and Levy, 1981). Because the brain changes in Alzheimer's disease are not uniform, but affect certain regions more than others, it might be expected that tissue density changes would also show regional variation. Such regional variations have indeed been reported (Bondareff, Baldy and Levy, 1981). However, despite these interesting leads, the overall contribution of CT scanning to the understanding of Alzheimer's disease has been disappointingly small.

The more recently developed technique of MRI yields similar information to CT scanning. However, it has the advantage of a much clearer resolution and does not involve exposing the patient to radiation. Because of the recent introduction of the technique, there has as yet been little application to Alzheimer's disease. Nevertheless, some early evidence shows that MRI can help distinguish Alzheimer's disease patients from normals as well as from patients with multi-infarct dementia (Besson *et al.*, 1983).

Of the existing brain imaging techniques, PET is likely to provide the most exciting discoveries. Like MRI, it is a quite recent development, but because of its complexity it is unlikely to be available outside specialised research centres for many years. PET involves injecting patients with a chemical which emits positrons. By selecting chemicals with particular biological functions, it is possible to trace various types of biochemical activity as they take place in the brain. Some research has involved tracing the use of glucose — this being the source of the brain's energy. Glucose utilisation has been found to be substantially reduced in Alzheimer's disease, but the reduction is not uniform over all regions, those involved in sensation and control of movement being least affected (Benson *et al.*, 1983; Foster *et al.*, 1984).

The most exciting application of PET will come with the use of positron-emitting chemicals which bind to particular neurotransmitter receptors. Some recent research with normal people has produced images reflecting the density of receptors for the neurotransmitters dopamine and serotonin (Wong *et al.*, 1984). This research found a decline with age in receptors for these neurotransmitters. If similar techniques can be developed for neurotransmitters like acetylcholine and somatostatin, which are affected in Alzheimer's disease, it may be possible to directly monitor the brain changes in Alzheimer's disease during life.

√ ARE THERE TWO TYPES OF ALZHEIMER'S DISEASE?

As pointed out in Chapter 1, it was once believed that Alzheimer's disease occurred only in people aged below 65 years and that it was separate from the senile dementia seen in the elderly. More recently, both have been referred to as Alzheimer's disease, because both involve dementia associated with plaques and tangles. However, there are some differences between those people whose Alzheimer's

31

disease comes early (before 70, say) and those who have the disease only very late in life (say, after 80). The existence of these differences has led to the suggestion that there are two distinct types of Alzheimer's disease, one of which tends to occur at a younger age than the other (Bondareff, 1983). However, the arbitrary age of 65, which was previously used to distinguish presenile Alzheimer's disease from senile dementia appears to be too low as a dividing point. Autopsy studies into Alzheimer's disease tend to divide the patients according to whether they died before or after the age of 79 or 80.

Early-onset Alzheimer's disease appears to be generally more severe than late-onset Alzheimer's disease. For example, the dementia progresses more rapidly, the loss of the enzyme CAT is more severe, and there is greater loss of cholinergic neurons from the basal forebrain. A recent study compared neurotransmitter deficiencies in early and late-onset cases and found that while the older cases had deficits involving acetylcholine and somatostatin, the younger cases had deficits in other neurotransmitters as well (Rossor *et al.*, 1984).

Clearly there are differences between early-onset and late-onset Alzheimer's disease, but do these justify the view that there are two types of the disorder? One way of demonstrating that there are two distinct types would be to find a qualitative difference between them — for example, a greater deficit in one neurotransmitter in early-onset cases as opposed to a greater deficit in a different neurotransmitter in late-onset cases. However, no such qualitative difference has yet been found; rather, early-onset cases simply seem to have greater deficits of the same kind or to be in a more severe stage of the disorder (Jorm, 1985). The more widespread neurotransmitter deficits of early-onset cases do not necessarily imply a qualitative difference. This difference can be readily explained in other ways. People who develop Alzheimer's disease at a later age are likely to die of other diseases to which the elderly are prone and so be in an earlier stage of the disease at the time of death. For example, in one Dutch study, people who developed Alzheimer's disease at the age of 70 or younger survived an average of 10 years after developing the disease. By contrast, people developing Alzheimer's at age 80 or over survived only 4½ years on average (Diesfeldt, van Houte and Moerkens, 1986). The longer survival of early-onset cases, together with their more rapid deterioration, ensure that they are in a more severe stage of the dementia at the point of death. If late-onset cases were to survive to a later stage, we might expect them to also develop widespread neurotransmitter deficits.

Another way of demonstrating distinct types would be to show that there is no gradual shading of one into the other, rather a natural break. Thus, if we were able to show that there is a large group of Alzheimer patients with a small degree of neuron loss from the basal forebrain and a second large group with massive loss, but very few with moderate loss, this would indicate a natural break between the two groups. However, again, no such evidence exists (Jorm, 1985). Rather, we seem to be dealing with a continuum ranging from rapidly advancing severe early-onset cases to more slowly advancing and less severe late-onset cases. Possible reasons for the greater severity of early-onset cases will be discussed in Chapters 6 and 7.

√ ALZHEIMER'S DISEASE AND NORMAL AGEING

Although Alzheimer's disease is often thought of as being a specific disease quite different from normal ageing, the differences between the two are largely a matter of degree. Most normal elderly people have plaques and tangles in their brains and show a loss of the enzyme CAT. However, these changes are greatly exaggerated in Alzheimer's disease and, in the later stages of the disorder, there may be other neurotransmitter changes as well. One way of accounting for these similarities is to propose a continuum, at one end of which is normal ageing and, at the other end, severe Alzheimer's disease. With age, people tend to move along the continuum, but some people move at a faster rate than others. Brain changes such as plaques, tangles and loss of CAT can take place up to a certain point without any major psychological consequences. But eventually the effects on memory, intelligence and personality are such that the individual's ability to cope with the demands of life is impaired. At this point, a person is regarded as demented and this dementia is ascribed to Alzheimer's disease. For people who move along the continuum at a faster rate, the onset of Alzheimer's disease will be more rapid. By contrast, for those moving at a slow rate, the onset of dementia will only be very late in life and the course will be slow. There will be some people whose progress along the continuum is so slow that they do not become demented, even if they reach extreme old age. The question of interest then becomes: why do some elderly people move along the continuum at a fast rate and others very slowly? This question is considered further in Chapters 6 and 7, but first we digress to discuss the cognitive effects of Alzheimer's disease.

5

Cognitive Deficits in Alzheimer's Disease

The term *cognitive deficit* refers to deficiencies in acquiring and manipulating knowledge. It thus includes problems of perception, attention, imagery, memory, language, and reasoning; in short, cognition embraces all aspects of human intelligence. Although people suffering from Alzheimer's disease have severe cognitive deficits, they are not equally deficient at all cognitive tasks. Particularly in the early stages of the disorder, some cognitive functions are more affected than others. However, in severe dementia all cognitive functions become greatly impaired. In this chapter we look specifically at the pattern of cognitive impairment in Alzheimer's disease.

MEMORY DEFICITS IN ALZHEIMER'S DISEASE

*Memory deficits are often one of the first noticed signs of Alzheimer's disease. However, human memory is not a unitary function. There are different kinds of memory and each of these involves several processes. One useful distinction is between *working memory* and *long-term memory*.

Working memory

Working memory (sometimes called primary or short-term memory) is used for temporary storage of information in everyday cognitive tasks and has a very limited capacity. To illustrate the role of working memory, try adding up the following numbers without using pen or paper: $9 + 8 + 4 + 11 + 6 =$? Most people do this task by adding 9 and 8 to get a subtotal of 17, then adding 4 to 17 to get a new subtotal of 21, adding 11 to 21, and so on. The particular subtotals generated along the way are only held in memory long enough to add on the next number and are then forgotten. Working memory is involved in retaining these subtotals. Another example of the use of working memory is in looking up an unfamiliar telephone number and then retaining it just long enough to be able to dial correctly. A temporary memory of small capacity is quite useful in such situations. There would be little point in retaining subtotals for more than a few seconds or in learning telephone numbers that need to be used only once. Working memory derives its name from its role as a sort of work space or mental scratch pad in more complex cognitive tasks such as doing arithmetic calculations or using the telephone. Information can be retained in working memory only for a matter of seconds unless it is actively refreshed by, say, mentally repeating it over and over.

Alzheimer's disease seems to involve some deficiency in working memory. Evidence for this comes from memory span tasks which assess the capacity of working memory. One commonly used type of memory span task gives people digits (numbers 0–9) at the rate of one every second. The number of digits is varied from short sequences, for example 3–9–5, up to quite long ones, for example, 4–6–9–3–2–5–8–6–1. The maximum number of digits a person can consistently hold in working memory is the digit span. Whereas normal elderly people can hold around six or seven digits in working memory, Alzheimer's disease patients with mild to moderate impairment can manage only around five digits (Kopelman, 1985; Nebes, Martin and Horn, 1984). This reduced memory span in Alzheimer's patients is also found when non-verbal working memory is assessed. For example, in one study, a tester showed some black blocks randomly fixed on a board which were tapped with a pen in a certain order. The patient than had to reproduce exactly the same patterns of taps. Memory span was measured by the largest number of blocks which could be tapped in the correct order. Even mildly impaired Alzheimer's patients were found to be poorer at this task and severe cases were greatly impaired (Corkin, 1982).

Once information is stored in working memory it is rapidly forgotten unless it can be refreshed by mental repetition. One way of testing the rate of forgetting from working memory is to give a small amount of information to be held (for example, three letters) and then prevent the person from refreshing them by requiring a distractor task to be carried out. Thus, the person might be told to

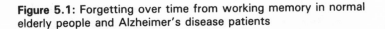

Figure 5.1: Forgetting over time from working memory in normal elderly people and Alzheimer's disease patients

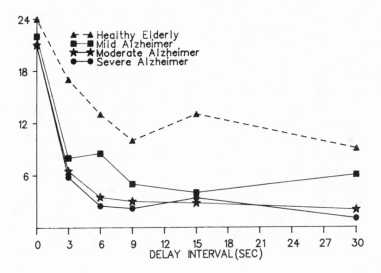

Source: adapted from Corkin (1982)

remember the letters G, P, B and then asked to count backwards from 973 for 10 seconds. After the 10 seconds is up they have to recall as many of the letters as possible. The amount of information lost shows how much forgetting has taken place over the 10 seconds. By testing forgetting many times over several different delays, it is possible to draw a graph of forgetting from working memory. Figure 5.1 shows such a graph. It can be seen that mild, moderate, and severe Alzheimer patients all show increased forgetting from working memory.

Long-term memory

Long-term memory is the more permanent kind of memory. In contrast to working memory it has a very large storage capacity and can hold information from minutes to decades. The operation of long-term memory involves three stages: *encoding, storage* and *retrieval*, which can be understood by analogy with the workings of a library.

When a new book comes into a library it must be catalogued — that is, the librarian must classify it by subject, title and author and place it on the appropriate shelf so that it can be found when needed. A book may sit on a shelf unused for many years and the ink may fade or the pages be eaten by insects. However, when it is needed by a reader, he or she will look up the title, author, or subject in the catalogue or scan the appropriate shelf to find it. If the book has been improperly catalogued or placed on the wrong shelf it will be difficult to find even though it is still held by the library. The process of cataloguing a book and placing it on an appropriate shelf is analogous to encoding it in long-term memory. During encoding, new information is interrelated with existing information to make it easy to retrieve later on. Books sitting on the shelves are analogous to storage in long-term memory. As with a library, information may be lost during storage through decay. The process of finding a book in a library is like retrieval from long-term memory. Often information which cannot be recalled is not lost, but simply cannot be retrieved because it was poorly encoded in the first place. Poor encoding is like poor cataloguing or mis-shelving a book in a library.

Encoding

We will now look at the evidence on the processes of encoding, storage and retrieval in the long-term memories of Alzheimer's disease patients. People with Alzheimer's disease appear to have difficulty encoding information properly. A good example of this comes from a study of Weingartner and his colleagues (1981). On three separate occasions, they gave normal elderly people and Alzheimer patients a list of words to remember. On one occasion, they had to remember 20 unrelated words. On another occasion the 20 words came from two broad categories (for instance, ten words were vegetables and ten were parts of the body). However, the words from the categories were all mixed together. Finally, they had to remember a list where the words were arranged together according to the category they were from. After a list of 20 words was presented one word at a time, the people had to recall as many of the words as they could in any order they liked. Normal people find lists of words which come from broad categories much easier to remember than unrelated words, even when the categories are all mixed up. This is because they organise the words into categories in their long-term memories and so find them easier to retrieve later on. Put another way, they use categories to help them encode the words in long-term memory. Weingartner *et al.* (1981) found, by

Figure 5.2: Alzheimer's disease patients have great difficulty recalling lists of words even when they are organised into categories

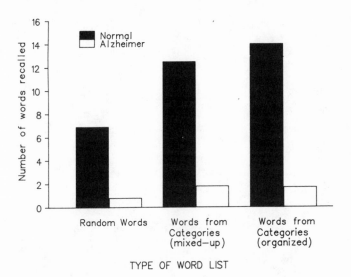

Source: adapted from Weingarter *et al.* (1981)

contrast, that Alzheimer patients are helped very little by having to learn words from only certain categories. Even when the words were presented for learning already organised into categories they gained very little benefit. These drastic results are shown in Figure 5.2. It thus appears that Alzheimer's disease patients have a major difficulty in effectively encoding new information in long-term memory, even when the information is organised to make this easy for them.

Storage

Although Alzheimer's disease involves major encoding deficiencies, long-term storage may be affected little if at all. That is, once information is in long-term memory it appears to stay there relatively well. A study by Kopelman (1985) illustrates the operation of long-term memory storage in Alzheimer patients. Kopelman recognised that loss of information from long-term memory is difficult to assess in demented people because their initial encoding of that information

Figure 5.3: Rate of forgetting from long-term memory in normals and Alzheimer patients

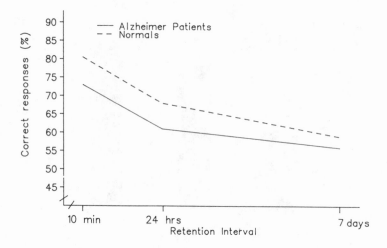

Source: adapted from Kopelman (1985)

will be worse. To overcome the problem he gave the demented patients much longer to learn the information. The exact task he used involved remembering pictures taken from magazines. Alzheimer patients were allowed to view each picture longer so that their initial memory was similar to that of the normals. Retention of the pictures was then measured by testing memory one day and then one week after initial learning. The patients had to pick out the original pictures from amongst a group of 'distractor' pictures. Surprisingly, Kopelman found that the forgetting rate for the Alzheimer patients was not much different from normals. As can be seen in Figure 5.3, although their 10 minute retention was a little poorer, the rate of forgetting was not greater thereafter. As Kopelman so aptly commented in his report on these findings, the problem is in getting information into long-term memory, but 'once accomplished the store does at least have a solid "floor"' (p. 538).

Retrieval

The final process in long-term memory is retrieval. Retrieval from long-term memory takes place in response to a *retrieval cue* — some aspect of the situation which gives a clue as to where the information is stored in long-term memory. In libraries, authors' names, titles, and subject headings are all retrieval cues for finding books. In long-term memory, retrieval can be relatively easy if the cue gives immediate access to the information, as in questions like: 'What is your name' or 'What season is it right now?'. However, sometimes the cues provided in the question are inadequate to retrieve the information. Thus, if we are asked: 'What was the name of your second grade teacher?', we might not be able to answer it at first because the cues provided by *second grade* and *teacher* are not suitable. In such cases, we can actively try to produce other cues which might lead the answer to 'pop out'. For example, we could form an image of the school, or the teacher's face, or the classroom, and one of these might be a sufficient cue to retrieve the teacher's name. This sort of active retrieval, where we have to work at finding answers by generating retrieval cues has been called *recollection* (Baddeley, 1982) and is a much more difficult process.

Recollection

Alzheimer's disease sufferers seem to have retrieval as well as encoding difficulties, particularly where the more difficult kind of retrieval we have termed *recollection* is involved. With simple sorts of retrieval, Alzheimer's disease patients do fairly well. For example, they can read single words aloud quite well (Nebes, Martin and Horn, 1984), suggesting that retrieval of word names using their printed forms as a cue is preserved. However, Alzheimer patients perform quite poorly at retrieval tasks which require them to list as many words as possible beginning with a certain letter (such as S) in 60 seconds (Miller, 1984) or to tell all the things they would do after getting up in the morning and before leaving the house (Weingartner *et al.*, 1983). In these situations it is not simply a matter of retrieving a single answer in response to a cue, but of generating suitable retrieval cues for oneself so as to produce as many answers as possible.

Interestingly, the retrieval of Alzheimer's disease patients can be improved somewhat by providing them with better cues. For example, E. Miller (1975) gave Alzheimer patients lists of ten words to learn. He found that their recall of these words was much worse than that of normal people. However, if he gave the patients the first letter of each word as a retrieval cue, their recall improved to the point where it was not much worse than normal. Similar results have been found by other researchers (Morris, Wheatley and Britton, 1983). It therefore seems that Alzheimer's disease patients have more stored in memory than their performance actually suggests. Because of their retrieval difficulties they are unable to locate all the information held in their memories unless specific retrieval cues are provided for them.

INTELLECTUAL DEFICITS IN ALZHEIMER'S DISEASE

Loss of intelligence invariably occurs in Alzheimer's disease, but in the early phases of the disorder, some intellectual skills decline more than others. Some idea of the aspects of intelligence which are most prone to decline can be gained by looking at scores on one widely used test of intelligence, the Wechsler Adult Intelligence Scale. The Wechsler scale consists of eleven separate tests of cognitive skills; six of these yield a measure of *verbal intelligence* and the other five *performance intelligence*. Verbal intelligence is measured by tests requiring a person to define the meanings of words, answer general knowledge questions, perform arithmetic calculations, hold digits in working memory, state how objects are alike (for example, *pear* and *banana*), and explain proverbs and social conventions. By contrast, performance intelligence tests require pictures to be arranged in order to tell a story, the missing parts of pictures to be found, blocks to be arranged to make patterns, jigsaw puzzles to be solved, and special symbols to be written as quickly as possible beside numbers. Although the verbal tests differ from the performance tests in that there is a greater involvement of language, another difference lies in the degree of novelty of the tests. The verbal tests tap the more practised aspects of intelligence and also those which are most directly improved by educational opportunities. The performance tests, however, involve largely unfamiliar problems of a sort less often encountered during schooling. Studies which have given the Wechsler scale to Alzheimer patients find that, although both components of intelligence are impaired, this is greater with performance intelligence than with verbal intelligence (Martin and Fedio, 1983; Moore and Wyke, 1984; Weingartner *et al.*, 1981).

Although global changes in intelligence are interesting, it is more useful to know about the specific intellectual skills which are impaired in Alzheimer's disease. As mentioned in the last chapter, cognitive skills controlled by the cortex are often specifically affected in the disorder. Indeed, some clinicians believe that these cortical cognitive impairments are so characteristic of Alzheimer's disease that it is possible to use them to differentiate it from certain other types of dementia (Cummings and Benson, 1983).

Language impairment

Severe language impairment, known as *aphasia*, is often found in Alzheimer's disease. However, the language impairment of Alzheimer's patients is not uniform; some functions are more affected than others.

One very basic aspect of language is the ability to name objects correctly. Alzheimer's disease patients have difficulty with finding the names of objects, particularly where the object is not a common one, and this difficulty becomes greater as the dementia progresses (Kirshner, Webb and Kelly, 1984). When Alzheimer patients make errors in naming objects they often give answers which are related in meaning to the correct answer (Martin and Fedio, 1983). For example, they may describe what the object does or where it can be found, give a word of similar meaning, substitute a more general category (such as 'vegetable' for asparagus), or name a related object ('mummy' for sphinx). Errors of this type indicate that Alzheimer's disease patients may suffer from a disruption in the organisation of word meanings in memory.

When their language is studied closely it is found to be rather empty and vague, perhaps because of the difficulty in retrieving word names and meanings from memory. Hier, Hagenlocker and Shindler (1985), for example, asked Alzheimer's disease patients to describe what they saw in a picture and found they tended to use more empty words, more pronouns in place of nouns, used prepositions inappropriately and made fewer relevant observations on the picture. The following example from a patient in this study clearly exhibits these characteristics; features of interest are printed in italics:

He almost fell [empty word]

Well, this *one* is drying what *she* had made drying the *stuff* [three empty words]

And this *one* almost fell down [empty word, repetition of earlier phrase]

And this *one* is holding that *he* should give *her something* and that was *it* [five empty words]

Right? [comment to examiner]

Water is going.

And *she has she has* got *this* [repetition of words, two empty words]

That is all [comment to examiner]

There is some cups.

43

I do not know if *they* cleaned *it* or not [two empty words, comment to examiner]

There is a window here.

You want the window [comment to examiner]

Did I give you this *one?* [empty word, comment to examiner]

Put *it* on the window [comment to examiner, empty word]

And *it* is a [empty word, incomplete thought]

They can close *it* and people cannot peek *it* [error in choice of preposition, three empty words]

Look in, right? [comment to examiner]

It is a window [repetition of earlier phrase]

But there is [incomplete thought]

(From Hier, Hagenlocker and Shindler, 1985, pp. 131–2, with minor changes to notes in brackets).

By contrast to these deficiencies, there is an aspect of language which is less affected in Alzheimer's disease. This aspect is *syntax* or the knowledge of how words are combined to make grammatically correct sentences. For example, the sentences from the patient quoted in the previous paragraph are basically grammatical, even though rather vague in meaning. It has been found that elderly dementia patients (probably with Alzheimer's disease) are relatively good at correcting syntactically incorrect sentences such as: *Write down it, He give me candy,* and *She called today, didn't her?* (Bayles and Boone, 1982).

Perceptual impairment

Although the basic processes of vision are unaffected in Alzheimer's disease (Moscovitch, 1982), there can often be a difficulty in recognising objects. This type of impairment, where objects are seen but not recognised correctly, is known as *agnosia*. With severe agnosia, even the faces of familiar people may not be recognised. However, problems of recognition are most apparent when an object cannot be clearly seen. Kirshner, Webb and Kelly (1984) investigated such problems by asking Alzheimer patients to name objects under varying degrees of perceptual difficulty. The clearest perceptual information was provided by showing actual objects; less information by showing photographs; less still by line drawings; and the least by 'masked' drawings in which a pattern of intersecting lines was superimposed on the drawings. Because of their difficulty

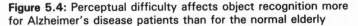

Figure 5.4: Perceptual difficulty affects object recognition more for Alzheimer's disease patients than for the normal elderly

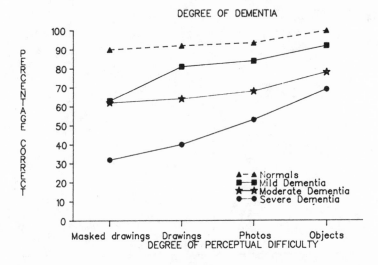

Source: adapted from Kirshner, Webb and Kelly (1984)

in retrieving object names from memory, Alzheimer patients would be expected to do poorly whatever the extent of perceptual information. However, if they have problems in perceptual recognition, they should also be adversely affected by lack of perceptual information. The results are shown in Figure 5.4. It can be seen that the Alzheimer's disease patients were worse overall because of naming impairment, but were also affected by the degree of perceptual information provided. The normal group, by contrast, was little affected by perceptual difficulty.

Visual-spatial impairment

Visual-spatial impairment involves difficulty in moving about according to some plan. When demented people become lost at the shops or have difficulty finding the way around their own house they are showing visual-spatial impairment. In the clinic such difficulties can be shown by having demented patients copy or produce spontaneous drawings. For example, Moore and Wyke (1984) asked fifteen

45

Figure 5.5: Left: spontaneous drawings of a cube by demented patients; Right: copies of a cube drawing by demented patients

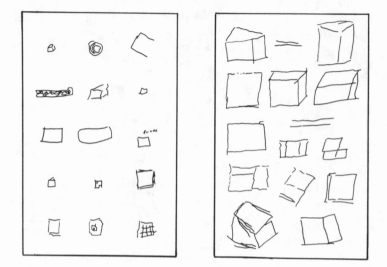

Source: Moore and Wyke (1984)

Alzheimer patients to do drawings of a house and cube. The resulting cube drawings are shown in the left half of Figure 5.5. The most notable differences from the drawings of normal individuals are that many essential features are left out and the drawings are small and cramped in appearance. When given a drawing and asked to copy it, the demented patients improved (see right half of Figure 5.5) in that more essential details were included and the drawings were larger, but the details were often positioned wrongly. Moore and Wyke thought the demented patients might be poor at copying because they focused attention on one feature of the drawing at a time and did not integrate the separate features into a coherent whole.

AUTOMATIC AND EFFORTFUL COGNITIVE PROCESSING IN ALZHEIMER'S DISEASE

Although in the severe stage of Alzheimer's disease there is global cognitive impairment, in the mild and moderate stages some skills are more impaired than others. Are there any common features to the skills which are impaired early compared to those which are resistant to decline? One suggestion is that *automatic* cognitive processes hold up relatively well while *effortful* or *controlled* processes decline early (Jorm, 1986a).

Effortful or controlled processes are those that require a person's attention. When a task requiring effortful processing is being carried out, it is difficult to perform another task at the same time without interference occurring. Effortful processing is involved with unfamiliar tasks or those which require the person to adapt to unpredictable circumstances. By contrast, automatic processing requires minimal attention and two automatic processes can be carried out simultaneously without interference. The advantage of automatic processing is that it allows predictable tasks to be carried out while leaving the person's attention free to handle novel situations. However, it cannot be used for novel or unpredictable situations. When a new task is encountered, the person's full attention is required and it feels effortful. However, if the task is predictable it will gradually become automatic with practice and attention can be diverted to other matters. Thus, the process of learning involves a gradual transition from effortful to automatic processing. To take a concrete situation, imagine a person having his or her first driving lesson. For the beginner it takes full concentration to keep the car on the road, to change gears, or to brake. If the instructor tries to carry on a conversation, it is impossible to attend to it and the driving simultaneously without one of them suffering. However, after years of practice, it is possible to drive over familiar routes while carrying on quite a deep conversation or listening intently to the radio. Changing gears and steering take place without effort or awareness. However, when driving through an unfamiliar town with busy traffic even experienced drivers will have to devote attention to the task and may find a passenger's conversation distracting.

The cognitive deficits seen in early Alzheimer's disease generally involve effortful processing. Effortful processing is involved when new information is encoded in memory. It is also involved in the sort of active retrieval from memory we have called *recollection* (see p. 41). However, storage of already encoded information involves no effort; nor does memory retrieval when clear retrieval cues are provided. These latter processes are little affected early in Alzheimer's disease.

With intellectual skills, effortful processing is more involved in performance intelligence than in verbal intelligence, because verbal skills are more familiar and practised. Again, it is performance intelligence which declines the most in the early stages of Alzheimer's disease. With language, the processing of meaning is effortful because it is unpredictable and requires conscious decision, whereas the rules of syntax are predictable and used unconsciously (Bayles and Boone, 1982). Similar arguments can be made in the areas of perceptual and visual-spatial disturbance. For example, Moore and Wyke (1984) explain the deficient figure copying of Alzheimer patients in terms of their inability to control their attention to focus on the figure as a whole rather than on its separate parts.

IMPORTANCE TO DIAGNOSIS

Research into cognitive deficits in Alzheimer's disease has barely begun, but may be of great practical significance if it can aid accurate and early diagnosis of the disorder. Certain diagnosis of Alzheimer's disease can presently be made only at autopsy, but it may be possible to diagnose the disorder with a fair degree of accuracy during the patient's life by assessing patterns of cognitive impairment. For example, in one recent study carried out in Finland an attempt was made to diagnose Alzheimer's disease during life by looking for cognitive deficits characteristic of the disorder and excluding other possible diseases. After these patients had died they were given an autopsy and the earlier diagnosis of Alzheimer's disease was found to be correct in over 80 per cent of cases (Sulkava et al., 1983).

If, in the future, useful treatments are developed to relieve the symptoms of Alzheimer's disease, it will be necessary to have accurate methods of diagnosis during life. Certain diagnosis at autopsy will simply be too late!

6

Risk Factors for Alzheimer's Disease

INTRODUCTION

Although plaques and tangles are a frequent occurrence in elderly people, in only a minority do they become so common as to produce dementia. There must be some characteristics which differentiate the minority who develop Alzheimer's disease from the majority who do not. Characteristics of this sort are known as *risk factors* because they indicate groups in the population who are at greatest risk for developing a disorder.

Many risk factors for Alzheimer's disease have been proposed, but not all have been consistently identified by different researchers. This chapter deals only with risk factors which have been confirmed in two or more independent studies. One can be fairly confident that these are genuine risk factors for Alzheimer's disease. To date, only five such risk factors have been identified. These are:

(1) Old age
(2) A family history of Alzheimer's disease
(3) Head trauma
(4) Down's syndrome, and
(5) A family history of Down's syndrome.

Although this list is small, it must be emphasised that research interest in risk factors for Alzheimer's disease has really begun only in the last few years. This area of research is growing so rapidly that many previously unknown risk factors may be discovered in the near future. The following sections look at each of the five confirmed risk factors in detail.

OLD AGE

Old age is undoubtedly the most important risk factor for Alzheimer's disease. As discussed in Chapter 4, autopsies show that the chances of having many plaques and tangles in the brain increase greatly with age. Another important piece of evidence for age as a risk factor comes from a study of the complete population of a community in southern Sweden from 1947 to 1972 (Hagnell *et al.*, 1983). By examining every member of this community at several points over this 25-year period, it was possible to detect all the new cases of dementia which arose. Figure 6.1 shows the percentage of people who developed Alzheimer's disease each year for different age groups. Nobody developed the disorder from ages 50 to 59, but thereafter the annual probability of developing it rose rapidly for both males and females. For people in their 80s, around 2 per cent of males and 3 per cent of females developed Alzheimer's disease each year. Strangely, in the 90s there was a drop-off in the development of new cases for males. This finding may be due to unreliability in the data, since only a very small number of males survive to this advanced age. However, it could be that those rare individuals who survive to be very old are a kind of elite whose chances of developing Alzheimer's disease are reduced. In fact, a study of senile plaques in relation to age has also reported a drop in occurrence in those aged over 90 (Matsuyama, 1983).

A FAMILY HISTORY OF ALZHEIMER'S DISEASE

To study the role of family history in Alzheimer's disease, it is necessary to find definite cases of Alzheimer's disease and then to investigate all relatives for the disorder. As simple as this may sound, there are some difficult problems involved because Alzheimer's disease is very much a disorder of the elderly. For instance, only relatives who have lived to old age will have had a chance to develop the disorder. Thus, it is possible to look for Alzheimer's disease in parents and siblings, but children of affected individuals are generally too young to have a chance to develop it. It is also necessary to carry out statistical adjustments to risk estimates to allow for relatives who may have developed Alzheimer's disease had they lived longer. Furthermore, investigating dementia in parents and siblings of Alzheimer cases necessarily involves studying individuals who may have died many

Figure 6.1: Chances of developing Alzheimer's disease rise with age

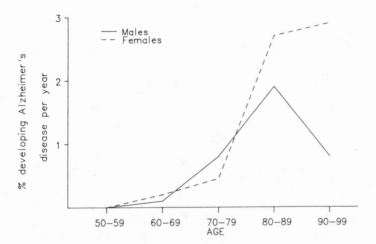

Source: based on data in Hagnell *et al.* (1983), for Lundby, Sweden, from 1947 to 1972

years ago. Because so little was known about Alzheimer's disease in the past, recollections about these relatives and even medical records may be unreliable.

Despite all these difficulties there is now good evidence that parents and siblings of Alzheimer's disease cases do have a greater risk of developing the disorder (Heston, 1981; Heyman *et al.*, 1983; Whalley *et al.*, 1982). Probably the most thorough study of family history is that of Heston (1981) in Minnesota, who studied the families of a large number of cases of autopsy-proven Alzheimer's disease. He found the risk to parents of these cases as being 15–23 per cent and the risk to siblings as 10–14 per cent. However, these general risk estimates are rather misleading because Heston found that the risk to relatives varies greatly depending on the age at which Alzheimer's disease began. Figure 6.2 shows the relationship between age of onset of Alzheimer cases and the risk to their siblings. There is a clear decrease in risk with later age of onset. Risk to parents shows a similar relationship. These findings are particularly interesting because early-onset Alzheimer's disease is known to be a more severe disorder with a faster course than late-onset Alzheimer disease (see Chapter 4). Putting these two pieces of

51

Figure 6.2: Risk to siblings by age of onset of Alzheimer's disease

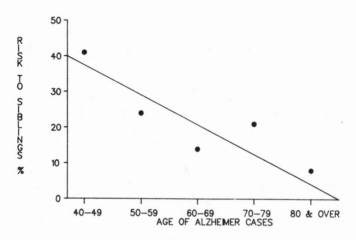

Source: adapted from Heston (1981)

information together, Alzheimer's disease may be more severe when it runs in families.

HEAD TRAUMA

It has been known for many years that professional boxers can develop a form of dementia. These boxers are often referred to as *punch-drunk*, although their disorder is technically known as *dementia pugilistica*. It is similar to Alzheimer's disease in that numerous neurofibrillary tangles are present. However, senile plaques are absent or scarce. Because the experience of boxers shows that trauma (physical injury) to the head can cause dementia, there has been a lot of recent interest in whether it could also predispose to Alzheimer's disease. Several studies have now shown that Alzheimer's disease sufferers are more likely to have experienced head trauma at some point in their lives (Heyman *et al.*, 1984; Amaducci *et al.*, 1985; Mortimer *et al.*, 1985).

In the first study of the issue, Heyman and his colleagues compared 40 cases of Alzheimer's disease with 80 people of the same age from the general community. They found that 15 per cent of the Alzheimer's disease patients had suffered previous head trauma, but only 4 per cent of the normal group. The patients in this study had early-onset Alzheimer's disease, but a later study by Mortimer and colleagues (1985) found the same result with a mixture of both early-onset and late-onset cases. Here 26 per cent of their Alzheimer cases were reported to have had previous head trauma, as against 15 per cent of people from the general community, and 5 per cent of non-demented hospital patients of the same age. In most cases where Alzheimer patients had suffered head trauma it was several decades before the onset of their dementia. The head trauma was generally due to a car accident and was serious enough to result in loss of consciousness. Unlike the situation with punch-drunk boxers where blows over many years have been sustained to the head, a single severe blow can predispose someone to Alzheimer's disease later in life. However, not everybody suffering such a severe blow will develop Alzheimer's disease. Head trauma increases the risk, but does not make the disease inevitable.

DOWN'S SYNDROME

Down's syndrome or *mongolism* is a disorder caused by an extra chromosome. It produces mental retardation as well as a host of bodily changes, the most noticeable of which are a fold over the corners of the eyes, a flat face and nose, and a large protruding tongue. Of greatest interest in the present context is that Down's cases seem to invariably develop plaques and tangles in their brains before their 40s. These changes are exceedingly rare in normal people of this age. Figure 6.3 shows the results of an autopsy study of 100 people with Down's syndrome. The incidence of plaques and tangles at death rises rapidly with age so that by early middle age all are affected.

Although Alzheimer-type changes are found in the brains of people with Down's syndrome, whether or not they show a dementia is often hard to say. By definition, dementia involves a loss of intelligence, so it is not clear how it might show in people who are mentally retarded to begin with. For the 49 individuals aged 31 and over represented in Figure 6.3, only thirteen showed clear signs of dementia before death even though all had plaques and tangles. Where dementia does occur in the mentally retarded it may not show in exactly the same way as in individuals of normal intelligence. From experience with several Down's syndrome cases, Heston (1984) has described the behavioural changes which take place as follows:

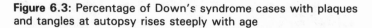

Figure 6.3: Percentage of Down's syndrome cases with plaques and tangles at autopsy rises steeply with age

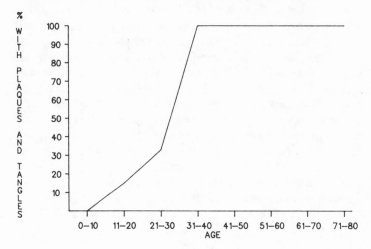

Source: based on data from Wisniewski *et al.*, (1985)

What occurs is that a typically energetic, happy-appearing, active person with Down's, who seems to enjoy his daily rounds of activities and recreations, especially simple games and music, begins to change. Less attention is given to hygiene; social exchanges become less spontaneous; basic skills, such as dressing, become less precise; names of attendants are apparently forgotten. Over a short time, months rather than years that similar changes require in [Alzheimer's disease], progression occurs to overt disorientation, often profound loss of weight and development of seizures, and, after becoming bedfast, to death (p. 289).

Although Down's syndrome is an uncommon disorder, sufferers are clearly a high-risk group for developing the brain changes characteristic of Alzheimer's disease. The reason for this strong association is presently unclear, but it may eventually provide some valuable clues to the causes of Alzheimer's disease.

A FAMILY HISTORY OF DOWN'S SYNDROME

In two studies, sufferers from Alzheimer's disease have been found to have an excess of Down's syndrome amongst family members, with several times the expected rate (Heston, 1982; Heyman *et al.*, 1983). However, because Down's syndrome births are a fairly rare occurrence (affecting about thirteen births in 10 000 in the United States), the incidence amongst relatives of Alzheimer's disease sufferers is still rather small and only becomes evident when a large group of relatives is studied. Furthermore, the excess of Down's syndrome in relatives has only been reported for cases which had an early onset. In the more common cases of later-onset Alzheimer's disease, there seems to be no excess of Down's syndrome in relatives.

To add further weight to the link between Alzheimer's disease and Down's syndrome, there are similarities in fingerprint patterns between sufferers from the two disorders. It has long been known that people with Down's syndrome have different fingerprint and handprint patterns from normals. However, Weinreb (1985) has reported that Alzheimer's disease patients show similar differences. Figure 6.4 shows the types of fingerprint patterns that can be found. Type C, the ulnar loop, is the pattern of which Alzheimer's disease patients had an excess. Whereas only 26 per cent of normal people had eight or more ulnar loops on their ten fingers, 72 per cent of Alzheimer's disease patients had this many. A more recent study has confirmed the finding that ulnar loops are more frequent in people with Alzheimer's disease, but only in early-onset cases (Seltzer and Sherwin, 1986). Later-onset cases did not show any difference from normals.

Fingerprint patterns are, of course, laid down before birth and are believed to be largely under genetic control. The association of early-onset Alzheimer's disease with a family history of dementia, a family history of Down's syndrome and differences in fingerprint patterns is all consistent with an important role for genetic factors in these cases.

COMMONLY BELIEVED RISK FACTORS FOR ALZHEIMER'S DISEASE

Although there are at present only five confirmed risk factors for Alzheimer's disease, there are several other factors which are

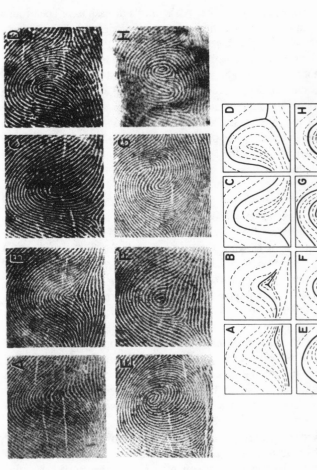

Figure 6.4: Types of finger-print patterns: A, simple arch; B, tented arch; C, ulnar loop; D, radial loop; E, central-simple whorl; F, central-pocket whorl; G, double-loop whorl; and H, accidental whorl

Source: Alter (1967)
Note: These prints are taken from the right hand. Ulnar and radial loops from the left hand will show the mirror-image of these patterns. With an ulnar loop, the pattern of flow comes from the direction of the little finger and loops back again in the same direction. For radial loops, the pattern of flow comes from the direction of the thumb and then loops back in this direction.

commonly believed by the public to confer risk for dementia in old age. The validity of these beliefs is worth considering.

Loss of former interests

Probably the most common belief is that old people become demented if they do not have lots of interests and remain mentally active. According to this view, the brain is an organ which will degenerate if not used. This belief is probably based on informal observations of old people who have lost their former interests and subsequently become demented. At this time, there has been no research on mental inactivity as a risk factor for Alzheimer's disease. Although it is possible that lack of mental activity produces dementia, it is more likely that this is in fact an early sign of the onset of dementia. It is quite common for demented people to show a reduction in range of activities and a loss of former interests as part of the early changes produced by their disorder.

Life stresses

A second factor often mentioned by the lay person is life stress. People who have a difficult, stressful life or have suffered from anxiety or depression are thought to be at greater risk. However, there is clear evidence that this factor does not increase the risk of developing Alzheimer's disease. Stressful life events and previous psychiatric disorders are no more common in the life histories of Alzheimer's disease sufferers than in normal elderly people (Heyman et al., 1984; French et al., 1985). However, depression is not infrequently found in the histories of Alzheimer's disease patients as an early symptom of the disease and could easily be mistakenly regarded as a cause of the disease by relatives.

Alcohol consumption

The final factor often mentioned by lay people is alcohol consumption. Alcohol is widely believed to lead to loss of brain cells and it is natural for people to wonder whether the cumulative effects could result in dementia. Certainly, overindulgence in the use of alcohol over a long period can lead to an alcoholic dementia. However, this type of dementia is rare, even among alcoholics, and is different from Alzheimer's disease. Among Alzheimer's disease sufferers, alcohol consumption has been found to be no greater than normal (Heyman *et al.*, 1984; French *et al.*, 1985), although (as will be discussed in Chapter 8) alcohol consumption could be a risk factor for the less common multi-infarct dementia.

IMPORTANCE OF RISK FACTORS FOR PREVENTION

While a full understanding of the causes of Alzheimer's disease and the development of an effective cure appear not to be even on the horizon, its occurrence may be controllable through preventive measures. Although prevention of Alzheimer's disease may seem a rather unattainable goal, this will not be the case if modifiable risk factors can be found. Many countries already have effective public health campaigns for reducing the incidence of diseases like cancer and heart disease which are based on persuading people to modify risk factors. A full understanding of the mechanisms of these diseases is not necessary for preventive approaches to work. Similarly, knowing that head trauma predisposes to Alzheimer's, we can attempt to prevent the disorder by reducing the incidence of head trauma. Much is already being done in some countries by requiring motorcyclists to wear helmets and motorists to wear seat belts. The other four confirmed risk factors — old age, a family history of Alzheimer's disease, Down's syndrome, and a family history of Down's syndrome — are unfortunately not modifiable. The challenge therefore is to discover additional risk factors which are modifiable by either legislation or persuading people to change their lifestyles. By this means a rational strategy for reducing the incidence of Alzheimer's disease can be developed even without a full understanding of its causes.

7

Theories of Alzheimer's Disease

The causes of Alzheimer's disease are unknown and are likely to remain so for many years. However, there have been several theories as to possible causes, some of which may eventually turn out to be close to the truth. In this chapter we will look at the evidence for and against three of these theories:

(1) Genes which predispose to Alzheimer's disease;
(2) Exposure to a toxic substance which affects brain function; and
(3) An infectious agent which invades the brain.

To be fully adequate any theory of the origins of Alzheimer's disease must explain why plaques and tangles develop in specific areas of the brain and why the cholinergic system is affected. It must also account for the five confirmed risk factors for Alzheimer's disease. Furthermore, such a theory needs to make new predictions about Alzheimer's disease which can be tested by researchers. In our current state of knowledge, these are tall orders to fill, and it is not surprising that no adequate theory of the causes of the disorder exists.

THE GENETIC THEORY

Some disorders (such as Huntington's disease) are transmitted from one generation to the next by a single defective gene. However, other disorders involve many genes. Studies of family histories can be used to work out possible genetic mechanisms. Disorders which involve a single gene show characteristic patterns of inheritance across generations. Alzheimer's disease does not seem to be transmitted by a single gene, except possibly in rare instances of families where there are many cases appearing at a fairly early age. To explain most cases of Alzheimer's disease by a genetic theory, it would be necessary to assume that many genes are involved (Wright and Whalley, 1984).

How might genes produce Alzheimer's disease? One view is that ageing is a genetically preprogrammed process. Just as genes act to turn on certain processes at specific times during a child's development, other genes act to shut down these processes in old age. There would be some genes which affect ageing of the brain, and a subgroup of these which specifically affect those brain processes responsible for memory and intelligence. Because of genetic differences between people, the timing of the shutdowns might vary from individual to individual. When the brain processes controlling cognitive functions shut down earlier than usual we label the individual as having Alzheimer's disease. This view explains the sharp rise in the prevalence of Alzheimer's disease with age.

The fact that people with Down's syndrome always develop the brain changes of Alzheimer's disease in middle age provides a valuable clue as to the nature of the genetic mechanisms which could be involved. Down's sufferers have an extra copy of one particular chromosome, labelled as *chromosome 21*. This extra chromosome means that Down's syndrome sufferers carry an extra supply of the genes on that chromosome. These extra genes may mean that certain essential chemicals within the body are overproduced. Heston (1984) has suggested that some product of the genes on chromosome 21 is important to the development of Alzheimer's disease.

A genetic theory may also be able to explain the family history of Down's syndrome among early-onset cases of Alzheimer's disease. In Chapter 2 we noted that the neurofibrillary tangles found in Alzheimer's disease could derive from normal structures in the nerve cell called *neurofilaments*. These neurofilaments, along with similar structures called *microtubules*, are important during the division of cells. There are two processes by which cells divide. The first occurs during growth when a single cell divides into two cells of the same type. The other kind of cell division occurs when sperm and ova are created for reproduction. In this situation, cells of 46 chromosomes divide to make sex cells with only 23 chromosomes. Sometimes this process goes wrong with the result that a sex cell might have an extra chromosome. Such cells are responsible for Down's syndrome. Heston and White (1978) have suggested that Down's syndrome and Alzheimer's disease could occur in the same families because of some basic defect of neurofilaments and microtubules. In the one case this defect affects cell division and creates Down's syndrome, and in the other produces neurofibrillary tangles within nerve cells. As intriguing as this idea is, it must be clearly recognised that it is very speculative at this stage of our knowledge.

The only risk factor not accounted for by a genetic theory is head trauma. This is clearly an environmental event. Although genetic factors are probably quite important in the development of Alzheimer's disease, they cannot be the only cause. There have been cases reported of identical twins (who have exactly the same genes) where one develops Alzheimer's disease and the other does not (Hunter, Dayan and Wilson, 1972). If genes were the only cause of Alzheimer's disease, identical twins should always develop the disorder together. There must therefore be environmental events which are important causes of Alzheimer's disease.

THE TOXIC-EXPOSURE THEORY

Alzheimer's disease could be due to some toxic substance which has a selective effect on certain regions of the brain which react by producing plaques and tangles. We know that toxic substances can have selective effects of this sort. In recent years it has been found that a chemical called MPTP (1-methyl-4-phenyl-1, 2, 3, 6-tetra hydropyridine) can produce Parkinson's disease by destroying nerve cells in a small region of the brain (Langston, 1985). This chemical can be absorbed through skin contact or inhalation. Could it be that there is a similar toxic substance which produces Alzheimer's disease? The most-discussed possibility has been aluminium.

During the 1960s it was observed that aluminium produced neurofibrillary tangles when injected into certain species of animals. Later, in the 1970s, it was reported that sufferers from Alzheimer's disease had aluminium in their brains, a finding not always confirmed by later researchers. However, not all nerve cells are affected by neurofibrillary tangles in Alzheimer's disease. When those cells specifically affected by neurofibrillary tangles were examined, they were found to have increased aluminium. By contrast, unaffected neurons did not (Perl and Brody, 1980).

Aluminium is a common substance in the earth's crust, so some degree of exposure is universal. Although it might be thought that aluminium cookware would increase intake, this is thought to be

61

only a minor source. Rather, antacids which contain aluminium are a major dietary source if taken over a long period (Shore and Wyatt, 1983). Another way aluminium can enter the body is through drinking water. Normally, aluminium is insoluble in water, but when the water is acidic it is dissolved more readily. In areas where acid rain occurs, the aluminium content of drinking water may increase greatly, leading to concern that it might produce a higher incidence of dementia (Pearce, 1985).

Despite all this circumstantial evidence, there are several reasons for being sceptical as to whether aluminium is a cause of Alzheimer's disease. Firstly, the neurofibrillary tangles produced in animals by aluminium are different in kind from those seen in Alzheimer's disease. However, animals do not naturally develop Alzheimer's disease in old age as humans do. Therefore, it is not possible to test theories that toxic exposures lead to Alzheimer's disease using animal subjects (which is perhaps fortunate for the animals concerned). Secondly, there is a type of dementia which occurs in kidney dialysis patients and is associated with high levels of aluminium. This concentration of aluminium is thought to be due to the presence of the metal in the large quantities of water needed during dialysis. However, the dementia found in these patients is not the same as Alzheimer's disease. Finally, it has been found that Alzheimer's disease patients are no more likely to have taken antacids containing aluminium than other people their age (Heyman et al., 1984).

Even though aluminium is probably not a cause of Alzheimer's disease, it may still be that patients with the disorder are vulnerable to aluminium in a way that other people are not. Perhaps nerve cells which are partially damaged by neurofibrillary tangles are more likely to accumulate aluminium. Although no evidence exists that aluminium intake makes Alzheimer's disease worse, some authorities have argued that it might be safer for Alzheimer's disease patients to avoid antacids which contain aluminium (Shore and Wyatt, 1983).

Even if aluminium turns out to be unrelated to Alzheimer's disease, there may yet be undiscovered toxic substances which produce the disorder. It has recently been reported that cases of early-onset Alzheimer's disease in Edinburgh are not randomly distributed throughout the city, but rather cluster in certain areas. The presence of some unknown toxic substance in those areas may explain this observation (Whalley and Holloway, 1985).

THE INFECTIOUS AGENT THEORY

The notion that Alzheimer's disease could be due to an infectious agent seems, at first glance, to be rather far fetched. However, there are two human diseases, similar in some ways to Alzheimer's disease, which are now known to be due to infectious agents. These diseases are kuru and Creutzfeldt–Jakob disease. Kuru is found amongst a tribe in a remote part of Papua New Guinea. Its major effect is uncoordination of muscular movement, but it also involves mild dementia. The traditional practice amongst this tribe was for the bodies of kinsmen to be eaten after death. The virus was transmitted by eating the brains of affected individuals. Since women and children most commonly ate the brains, they were most likely to develop kuru. Now that cannibalism has stopped, the disease is disappearing.

Creutzfeldt–Jakob disease occurs worldwide and is quite rare. It most often occurs in the elderly and involves a rapidly progressive dementia with death generally following within a year of onset. This disease has now been transmitted to a number of animal species, showing that some sort of infection is involved. There have also been cases of documented infection in humans. These have occurred through corneas transplanted from affected individuals and, in one case, from the use of a brain electrode which had previously been used on a sufferer. More recently, there has been concern that growth hormone derived from human pituitary glands after death can produce the disease.

Unconventional agents or prions

The agents that produce kuru and Creutzfeldt–Jakob disease are somewhat like viruses, but have a number of properties which differentiate them from previously known viruses. One of their most interesting properties is that they have long incubation periods, often of years or decades. Because of their differences from normal viruses they have been called *unconventional viruses* (Gajdusek, 1977) or *prions* (Prusiner, 1982). There has been much interest in whether Alzheimer's disease could also be due to one of these unconventional viruses. A demonstration that Alzheimer's disease could be transmitted to experimental animals would provide strong evidence that an infectious agent is involved. Many attempts have been made to do this by injecting animals with extracts from the

63

brains of affected humans, but they have so far been unsuccessful. These unsuccessful attempts may mean that an unconventional virus is not involved in Alzheimer's disease. However, there are other possible explanations. The infectious agent may only have its effects on humans, or perhaps the incubation period is so long that animals do not live long enough to show the disease (Prusiner, 1984). There is also as yet no evidence that Alzheimer's disease is transmitted between humans through intimate contact. If an unconventional virus is involved it is obviously not easily communicated to others.

The infectious agent theory does account for several of the risk factors for Alzheimer's disease. The fact that the disorder occurs in old age would be explained by the long incubation period of unconventional viruses. Only the elderly might have lived long enough to show the effects of an infection which is possibly present in many people. The family histories of Alzheimer's disease patients would be explained by transmission of the unconventional virus between family members. Similar family histories have been reported for Creutzfeldt–Jakob disease. Another risk factor to be explained is Down's syndrome. Down's syndrome sufferers are especially susceptible to conventional infections and it has been suggested that their condition may aid an unconventional virus to enter the brain and produce plaques and tangles (Wisniewski, Wisniewski and Wen, 1985).

Amyloid

Using the unconventional virus theory as a framework, Prusiner (1984) has given an unusual explanation of the abnormal protein called *amyloid* which is found at the core of senile plaques. He speculated that amyloid is actually an accumulation of the unconventional viruses. There is as yet no evidence to support this speculative account. Another interesting speculation involving the virus theory is that neurofibrillary tangles are produced by the presence of the virus. If this is so, then by finding the starting point of tangles in the brain during Alzheimer's disease, it may be possible to locate where the virus enters. By studying people who died in their late 50s and early 60s and were beginning to show tangles, Ulrich (1985) was able to narrow the possibilities down to the region of the nasal passage and pharynx. He speculated that a virus could spread from there along nerve pathways to the brain.

ARE THERE SEVERAL CAUSES OF ALZHEIMER'S DISEASE

Although we have looked at the genetic, toxic exposure, and infectious agent theories as though they were competing rivals, it is possible that more than one of them contains some truth. There could be several causes which act through some common mechanism to produce Alzheimer's disease. For example, several factors might cause certain critical nerve cells to die or might disrupt the blood–brain barrier, a membrane which protects the brain from many chemicals in the blood-stream.

Another possibility is that two or more of these potential causes must be present together to produce Alzheimer's disease. For example, certain genes might make people more susceptible to toxic exposures or viruses which then produce the disorder. In such a situation, neither factor in itself would be enough to cause the disorder, but in combination they would do so.

8

Multi-infarct Dementia

After Alzheimer's disease, multi-infarct dementia is the most common type of dementia in the elderly. However, it has not been the subject of the same sort of intensive research effort as Alzheimer's disease in recent years, with the consequence that much less is known about it.

This type of dementia is due to several strokes or *infarcts*, hence the term *multi-infarct dementia* (Hachinski, Lassen and Marshall, 1974). In a stroke there is a blockage of an artery supplying blood to part of the brain by, say, a blood clot. The lack of blood may lead to death of the nerve cells in that region. Such blockages occur more readily when there is *atherosclerosis*, a condition in which fatty deposits line the walls of blood vessels and cause narrowing. Of course, strokes do not always lead to dementia. Most often they produce quite specific deficits, the nature of which depends on the region of the brain affected. A person may even suffer several strokes without becoming demented (Ladurner, Iliff and Lechner, 1982). However, with the appropriate site and size of damage to the brain, a series of strokes can produce a general decline in cognitive skills.

PROBLEMS IN DIAGNOSING MULTI-INFARCT DEMENTIA

Multi-infarct dementia is hard to clearly differentiate from Alzheimer's disease while a person is still alive. Only after death can the infarcts in the brain be observed with certainty. Although multi-infarct dementia cannot be definitely diagnosed during life, there are some features which are more likely to be found in multi-infarct dementia than in Alzheimer's disease and other dementias. By taking

66

many of these weakly differentiating features together, it is possible to get an indication of whether a demented person is more likely to be suffering from multi-infarct dementia or some other disorder such as Alzheimer's disease. The most popular method of attempting a differentiation is by using the Ischaemic Score developed by Hachinski and his colleagues (1975). *Ischaemia* is a term used to describe a loss of blood supply to an area of the body, such as due to blockage in an artery. The Ischaemic Score is derived by looking for the features shown in Table 8.1. Important features are given a score of 2, and less important features a score of 1. Ischaemic Scores can vary between 0 and 18. People scoring 4 and below are regarded as unlikely to have multi-infarct dementia, while those scoring 7 and above are probable cases of the disorder. Scores of 5 and 6 are uncertain.

To find out whether the Ischaemic Score can successfully differentiate multi-infarct dementia from Alzheimer's disease and other dementias, there have been studies comparing its diagnoses during life with those made at autopsy. These studies have shown that the Ischaemic Score can differentiate multi-infarct dementia from other dementias to a large extent, but it is imperfect. A person with a *low* Ischaemic Score is unlikely to have multi-infarct dementia. Someone could not suffer strokes without them producing many of the features shown in Table 8.1. However, a person with a *high* Ischaemic Score does not necessarily have multi-infarct dementia (Liston and LaRue, 1983). For example, a person with a mixture of Alzheimer's disease and multi-infarct dementia will get a high score, as will a person with Alzheimer's disease together with strokes which have no connection with the dementia.

The problems in using the Ischaemic Score for diagnosis are not completely solved by modern computer-based techniques such as the CT scan which can provide images of the brain. CT scans will not show up small strokes called *lacunes*. These are strokes 2–15 mm in diameter which leave small holes behind as they heal. Lacunes are found deep in the brain and are believed by some authorities (such as Hachinski, Lassen and Marshall, 1974) to be an important cause of multi-infarct dementia.

Recently, there has been interest in using the level of *high density lipoprotein cholesterol* (or HDLC for short) in the blood as an aid to the diagnosis of multi-infarct dementia. HDLC is believed to play a role in taking cholesterol from body tissues to the liver where it is broken down (Miller and Miller, 1975). It is well known that a raised level of cholesterol is associated with atherosclerosis and the

67

Table 8.1: Ischaemic Score with brief explanations of features

Feature	Score	Explanation
Abrupt onset	2	Rather than a gradual cognitive decline over several years, there is a relatively sudden loss of cognitive skills.
Stepwise deterioration	1	After a stroke there will be a drop in function, followed by a stable period until the next stroke.
Fluctuating course	2	Immediately after a stroke there is a drop in function and afterwards a gradual improvement which does not, however, bring the person back to his or her previous level.
Nocturnal confusion	1	The person may become disoriented and wander at night.
Relative preservation of personality	1	There is less likely to be the apathy and emotional flatness often seen in Alzheimer's disease.
Depression	1	Despondency and pessimism may occur.
Somatic complaints	1	This includes complaints such as headaches, giddiness, blackouts, palpitations, ringing in the ears.
Emotional incontinence	1	If the person has even minimal cause to cry or laugh, it may be difficult to control.
History of hypertension	1	The person has had high blood pressure in the past.
History of strokes	2	The person has had strokes in the past.
Evidence of associated atherosclerosis	1	Signs of atherosclerosis can be observed in arteries outside the brain, such as at the back of the eye, the carotids, or the arteries to the legs or heart.
Focal neurological symptoms	2	The person reports impairment of vision, numbness or weakness in the face or a limb.
Focal neurological signs	2	*Specific* abnormalities with memory, language, perception, reading, control of movement, sensation, or reflexes can be observed.

Source: Hachinski *et al.*, 1975

action of HDLC is to reduce cholesterol. We might therefore expect that people with multi-infarct dementia would have less HDLC. This has indeed been found and it has been proposed that HDLC level could be used to differentiate multi-infarct dementia from Alzheimer's disease (Muckle and Roy, 1985). However, there is considerable overlap between the two disorders in HDLC levels, making it unsuitable as a diagnostic test on its own (Erkinjuntti, Sulkava and Tilvis, 1985). Another complication is that HDLC levels are affected by physical activity, so that bedridden demented patients have much lower levels than those who are active (Zanetti et al., 1985). Despite these difficulties, HDLC levels might be a useful aid in diagnosis when used with other tools such as the Ischaemic Score and CT scan.

POSSIBLE RISK FACTORS FOR MULTI-INFARCT DEMENTIA

Because so little research has been done on the topic, there are no risk factors for multi-infarct dementia about which we can be very confident. However, to date, six possible risk factors have been suggested. These are: old age, a family history of multi-infarct dementia, high blood pressure, smoking, drinking alcohol, and (rather incredibly) living in Japan. We could also include low HDLC levels (discussed in the previous section) as an additional risk factor.

Old age

As with Alzheimer's disease, the incidence of multi-infarct dementia rises sharply in old age. A study of the population of an area in southern Sweden found that, amongst people in their 50s, only about one in 4000 developed multi-infarct dementia each year. However, the chances of developing multi-infarct dementia rose to one in 60 per year for people in their 80s (Hagnell et al., 1983). As with Alzheimer's disease, there may be some slight fall-off in the incidence amongst those rare individuals who survive past 90.

Family history

The parents and siblings of people with multi-infarct dementia have a greater risk of developing the disorder themselves (Åkesson,

1969). Of greater interest would be to know the risk to children whose parents were affected. However, there is no information available on this topic because it would require waiting for the younger generation to become old before the risks could be calculated.

High blood pressure

Not all stroke victims develop dementia. A comparison between stroke patients with and without dementia revealed that high blood pressure was the main difference between them. Whereas 68 per cent of stroke patients with dementia were found to have high blood pressure, only 23 per cent of those without dementia had high blood pressure (Ladurner, Iliff and Lechner, 1982). High blood pressure is important in producing lacunes, the small strokes deep within the brain.

Smoking and alcohol

An Italian study comparing cases of multi-infarct dementia to normal elderly people found that they were more likely to be smokers and drinkers (Pinessi et al., 1983). However, these were weaker risk factors than high blood pressure. By contrast, this same study found smoking and drinking to be unrelated to Alzheimer's disease.

Living in Japan

Although multi-infarct dementia has been consistently reported as being less common than Alzheimer's disease by researchers in Western Europe and North America, Japanese researchers have reported that it is the more common type of dementia in their country (Karasawa, Kawashima and Kasahara, 1982; Hasegawa 1984). Unfortunately, all the available evidence is based on diagnosis while patients are still alive. Only with post-mortem diagnosis could we be certain that multi-infarct dementia is really more common in Japan. It might be that Japanese physicians diagnose multi-infarct dementia differently from physicians in the West. However, there is another piece of evidence that adds considerable credence to the Japanese reports. Stroke, which is the cause of multi-infarct dementia, is much more common in Japan. A study coordinated by the World Health Organization, using identical diagnostic methods across countries, found much higher rates of strokes in Japan compared to ten other countries (Aho *et al.*, 1980). Similarly, a study comparing the health of Japanese men living in Japan, Hawaii and California found that stroke was more common amongst those living in Japan (Kagan *et al.*, 1976). The reasons for this interesting difference are unknown. Perhaps it relates to high salt levels in the Japanese diet, since salt is known to raise blood pressure and high blood pressure predisposes to stroke.

PREVENTION OF MULTI-INFARCT DEMENTIA

Many of the possible risk factors for multi-infarct dementia can be modified. The health risks of high blood pressure, smoking and drinking alcohol are well known. We would expect that changes in risk factors might reduce the incidence of multi-infarct dementia. In fact, there is now good evidence from many countries that the incidence of stroke is declining (see, for example, Prineas, 1971; Garraway *et al.*, 1979; Ueda *et al.*, 1981). Figure 8.1 shows one set

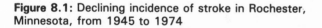

Figure 8.1: Declining incidence of stroke in Rochester, Minnesota, from 1945 to 1974

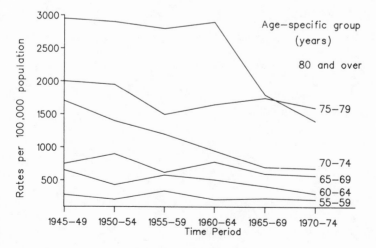

Source: adapted from Garraway *et al.* (1979)

71

of figures from the United States. This declining trend has been going on since the end of the Second World War and appears to be continuing. No one knows for sure why the decline has occurred. It could be because high blood pressure is now usually treated, or because of health warnings against smoking and high cholesterol diets. Whatever the reason, it is to be hoped that it will also affect the incidence of multi-infarct dementia.

9

Cognitive Deficit in the Depressed Elderly

In this chapter we leave senile dementia for a time and look at a quite different disorder — depression. The principal symptom of depression is a major change in mood which might be described as sad, blue, hopeless, low, down in the dumps, or irritable. In addition, a depressed person may show other symptoms such as loss of interest in activities which were previously pleasurable, poor appetite, sleeping difficulties, slowed movements, restlessness, fatigue, feelings of worthlessness or guilt, complaints of difficulty in concentration, and thoughts of death or suicide. Generally, only some of these symptoms will be seen in a particular case.

Depression is of particular interest in the present context because, in some cases, it may be confused with senile dementia. For example, a British study of patients admitted to hospital for dementia found 8 per cent to be cases of depression (Marsden and Harrison, 1972), while a similar Australian study found 5 per cent to be suffering from depression (Smith and Kiloh, 1981).

MEMORY COMPLAINTS IN DEPRESSION

One reason for confusing depression with dementia is that depressed people often complain of having a poor memory. Interestingly, though, there is little relationship between complaints about memory problems and actual impairment as revealed by memory tests. In fact, memory complaint may be accompanied by quite good memory performance. For example, in one study (Kahn et al., 1975), middle-aged and elderly psychiatric patients and their relatives were interviewed about their memories. They were asked 'Do you have any trouble with your memory?' and, if they did, to rate how severe it was. At the same time they were given some memory tests together with tests sensitive to brain impairment. Figure 9.1 shows the results. Note that depressed people complained that their memories were poor irrespective of whether they really had a poor memory or not. In fact, depressed people complained even more than non-depressed people who really had substantial memory impairment. The clear conclusion is that complaints of a poor memory should not be regarded as a symptom of dementia, but rather as a possible indicator of depressed mood.

COGNITIVE DEFICIT IN DEPRESSION

Even though depression may be accompanied by exaggerated memory complaints, there is now substantial evidence that depressed people can have impairments on tests of memory and intelligence (W.R. Miller, 1975). Such impairments can be found at all ages, but in the elderly they may be so severe as to lead to a mistaken diagnosis of dementia. Described below is such a case (Kiloh, 1961, pp. 341-2)

M.A.S. aged 52, a woman of adequate personality and normally bright and cheerful, had for two years been irritable, experiencing dizzy attacks, headaches and tinnitus. She admitted to a degree of depression and was concerned about the occurrence of nightmares. Her appetite had been poor and she had lost one stone in weight. Of all her symptoms, she placed most emphasis on the fact that her memory was failing, and that she could not remember where she had put things. Her daughter confirmed these statements and said that the patient did 'funny things' in the house, such as going to the coalshed when she intended to go to the pantry.

In hospital she showed a fluctuating mild depression but initially the most striking defects were in the field of memory and there was some inaccuracy of orientation in time. There was no suggestion of personality deterioration and there were no abnormal physical signs. It was felt that an early presenile dementia was the probable diagnosis. All investigations, including electroencephalography, proved normal. She was given imipramine in view of her depressive symptoms and after 10 days she showed considerable improvement. She was able to answer simple problems quickly and accurately, to interpret proverbs and she now

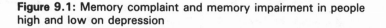

Figure 9.1: Memory complaint and memory impairment in people high and low on depression

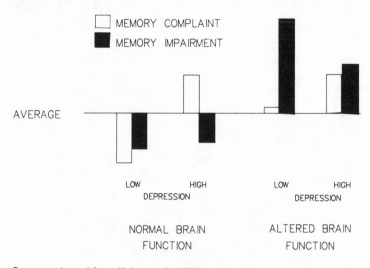

Source: adapted from Kahn *et al.* (1975)

showed a fair range of general information. Four weeks after discharge from hospital there was a mild but transient relapse. When last seen six months later she remained well. There was no longer any doubt that this was a case of mild endogenous depression; the possibility of a presenile dementia was discounted.

The effects of depression on cognitive function are clearly seen in a study which gave a test of cognitive function called the *Mini-Mental State Examination* to seriously depressed people of various ages (McHugh and Folstein, 1979). The Mini-Mental State has a series of questions like: 'What is the year?'; 'Write any complete sentence on a piece of paper for me'; and 'Spell WORLD backwards'. People are scored for number correct out of 30, with a score of 23 or less indicating cognitive impairment. Figure 9.2 relates the Mini-Mental State scores of the depressed people to their ages. It can be seen that some severely depressed people over 60 show a cognitive deficit, whereas none do at younger ages.

When depressed elderly people have such severe cognitive deficits it is not surprising that they can be mistakenly diagnosed as having senile dementia. In some cases, the degree of cognitive

Figure 9.2: Mini-Mental State scores of depressed patients of different ages. Each dot represents one person. The dashed line at a score of 24 represents the borderline for normal cognitive function

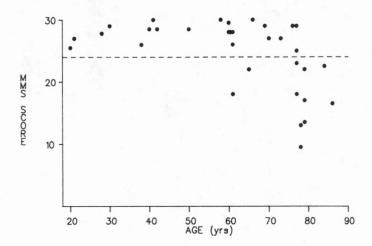

Source: adapted from McHugh and Folstein (1979)

impairment can be greater than that found in Alzheimer's disease. As an example, Figure 9.3 shows the Mini-Mental State scores of 16 cases of Alzheimer's disease compared to 24 elderly cases of severe depression. Although many of the depressed elderly have normal cognitive performance, some are worse than the Alzheimer cases.

It is very important that a correct diagnosis be made when depression is producing the cognitive impairment, because this disorder can often be successfully treated. By contrast, Alzheimer's disease and multi-infarct dementia have virtually no prospect for improvement. Figure 9.4 shows the results of treatment on the Mini-Mental State scores of ten elderly depressives. Although some are still cognitively impaired after treatment, others show normal cognitive function. However when Alzheimer's disease patients are simply retested on the Mini-Mental State after an equivalent period of time there is little change.

Figure 9.3: Mini-Mental State scores of depressed elderly patients and Alzheimer's disease patients

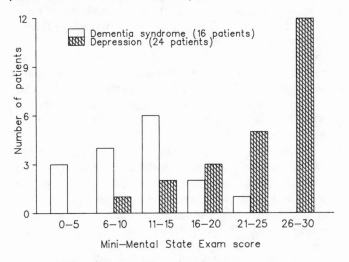

Source: adapted from McHugh and Folstein (1979)

Figure 9.4: Mini-Mental State scores of depressed patients who had cognitive impairment improve after treatment. By contrast, Alzheimer's disease patients show little change when retested after a similar period of time

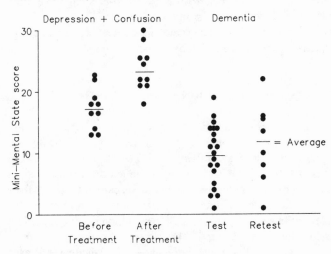

Source: adapted from McHugh and Folstein (1979)

POSSIBLE ORIGINS OF THE COGNITIVE DEFICIT

The reason for the cognitive deficit seen in depressed elderly people is still a matter of dispute. There are basically two views. The first is that the problem is motivational. Depressed people characteristically show a lack of interest in activities which would normally motivate them. This lack of interest could carry over to cognitive tasks, so that they do poorly through lack of effort. Those who take the view that the cognitive deficit is a motivational problem often refer to the disorder as *depressive pseudodementia* (Kiloh, 1961), implying that the dementia is not a real one.

The opposing view is that depression gives rise to a true dementia due to a brain disorder which just happens to be reversible with appropriate treatment. Those who advocate this view have referred to the disorder as the *dementia syndrome of depression* (Folstein and McHugh, 1978). One theory to explain this depressive dementia is that the brain changes in ageing combine with those in depression to have a major effect on cognitive function. Depression is believed by some authorities to involve a disturbance of the system of nerve cells which use *noradrenaline* as a neurotransmitter. These nerve cells play an important role in mood and may also have a role in memory. In young people, this neurotransmitter disturbance primarily affects mood and has only a small effect on cognition. However, in elderly people who have already lost neurons through ageing the noradrenaline disturbance greatly affects cognitive function as well as mood (Folstein and McHugh, 1978). As yet, there is not enough evidence to support either this view or the alternative motivational theory (Jorm, 1986b).

DISTINGUISHING DEPRESSION FROM DEMENTIA

Because the cognitive deficit in depression can be successfully treated, it is important for it to be correctly diagnosed. Unfortunately, there is no sure way of doing this. One idea is that depression produces a different type of cognitive deficit from that seen in dementia. For example, Alzheimer's disease often involves cognitive deficits due to impaired functioning of the cortex (for example, deficits of language and the recognition of objects), while depression does not (Caine, 1981). However, depression is most likely to be confused with the early stages of Alzheimer's disease when the cortical cognitive deficits are seldom present. They are therefore not a useful diagnostic sign in most cases. Another proposal is that depressed patients are more likely to give 'don't know' answers during cognitive tests, presumably because they are less motivated, whereas demented patients are more likely to give an incorrect answer (Wells, 1979). Unfortunately, recent research has shown that depressed elderly patients are no more likely to say 'I don't know' to questions than demented patients (Young, Manley and Alexopoulos, 1985).

A better approach to diagnosis may be to look closely for symptoms of depression in patients suspected of dementia. For example, a recent American study (Rabins, Merchant and Nestadt, 1984) compared the characteristics of patients who were demented with those who were depressed and had cognitive impairment. They found five characteristics which distinguished the depressed group:

(1) Onset of the disorder was more likely to have been recent (a matter of months rather than years);
(2) They were more likely to have suffered from depression previously;
(3) They currently had depressed mood;
(4) They tended to have irrational beliefs that they were physically ill, that their situation was hopeless, or that they were to blame for their predicament; and
(5) They were more likely to have a disturbed appetite.

Even though a close look for such symptoms of depression is useful, it may not succeed in diagnosing all cases correctly. An important reason is that demented patients often show signs of depression as part of their disorder. In one study, 23 per cent of demented patients were also depressed (Reifler, Larson and Hanley, 1982). Such patients will show signs of both dementia and depression, but their cognitive impairment will not be due to the depression.

RISK FACTORS FOR DEPRESSION IN OLD AGE

Elderly people who become depressed have been found to differ in a number of ways from other people their age. Table 9.1 shows some results from an important British study which compared depressed elderly patients with normal people of the same age drawn from the general community (Murphy, 1982). The depressed patients were more likely to have experienced severely adverse life events in the

Table 9.1: Frequency of adverse circumstances amongst depressed and normal elderly people

	Depressed(%)	Normal(%)
Severe life events in previous year	48	23
Major social difficulties	42	19
Chronic poor physical health	39	26

year preceding their depression. Such events included death or separation from a loved one, a life-threatening illness in someone close, or a physical illness in the depressed person. They were also more likely to have major social difficulties, lasting two years or more, before the onset of the depression. The major social difficulties included poor health of someone close, problems with housing, and difficulties in family or marital relationships. Personal health difficulties were also an important factor in those who became depressed. These physical health difficulties ranged across a spectrum of conditions, so it is unlikely that the illnesses had some direct biological effect in causing depression. Rather, major illness in the elderly is frequently a sign of approaching death and there is usually no hope that the condition will improve. Thus, physical ill-health implies a hopeless situation and thereby provokes depression.

Not all elderly people who experienced adverse circumstances became depressed. Those who were most vulnerable to the effects of such circumstances were the elderly who lacked an intimate confiding relationship. Such a relationship seemed to act as a buffer against adversity. However, intermittent intimate contact seemed to be as protective as full-time contact. Even those elderly people who saw a confidante such as a child or a brother or sister only every few weeks were buffered from the effects of adversity. Where social isolation existed it often seemed to be a consequence of a lifelong pattern of avoiding close relationships rather than a particular circumstance of old age.

Although social circumstances seem to be important risk factors for depression in old age, biological factors are important too. Some of the depressed elderly experience no adverse circumstances preceding their depression. These depressions which appear unexpectedly may be due to a biological predisposition to depression. Studies of depression in families show that close relatives of severely depressed patients have an increased risk of becoming depressed themselves. Also, studies of identical twins have shown that if one suffers depression the other twin is likely to as well. By contrast, with fraternal twins, who are only as genetically alike as normal brothers or sisters, there is a lower chance of one twin suffering from depression if the other does. However, for people who become depressed for the first time late in life the risk to relatives is much lower than with cases of depression occurring at a younger age (Slater and Cowie, 1971). Genetic factors may therefore be less important to the development of depression in the elderly than in the young.

An important role of research on risk factors is to give a basis for preventive action. Generally speaking, adverse life events, major social difficulties, and chronic ill-health in the elderly are not readily modified. The only exceptions would be in areas like housing difficulties and financial loss. However, the buffering effect of an intimate relationship, even if only occasional contact is involved, provides encouragement that some preventive action is possible.

10

Delirium

This chapter examines a disorder often associated with dementia and sometimes confused with it. This disorder is *delirium*, also sometimes referred to as an *acute confusional state*. Delirium is like dementia in that it involves significant cognitive impairment. However, whereas dementia is generally an irreversible condition involving progressive deterioration, delirium is a temporary state lasting only a matter of days or weeks. Although there has been an explosion of knowledge about dementia in recent years, delirium is still a poorly understood condition, despite its being quite common.

FEATURES OF DELIRIUM

According to the widely used diagnostic criteria of the American Psychiatric Association (1980), delirium involves the following features:

(1) *Consciousness is clouded* in that during delirium a person is not clearly aware of his or her environment. They have difficulty in attending to important features and are easily distracted by unimportant ones. It may be difficult to carry on a meaningful conversation with a delirious person because their attention will wander.

(2) *There is disorientation and impairment of memory.* The correct day, month, year and place will generally not be known. The delirious person will have difficulties in remembering recent experiences as well as in new learning. Because of these features the delirious person is often described as 'confused'.

(3) *Delirium develops rapidly* (in hours or days) and fluctuates in

severity over the course of a day. In this regard, delirium is clearly different from dementia, which generally develops gradually over months or years.

(4) *The condition is caused by some organic factor* such as an infection, recovery from a surgical operation, or the adverse effects of prescribed drugs.

(5) In addition, there may be some of the following:

   (a) *Perception may be disturbed.* During delirium a person will sometimes see things that are not there (for example, people in the room watching him) or will misinterpret what is seen (for example, a hospital room may be seen as the office where the person worked decades ago). These unreal perceptions are sometimes of a threatening nature and provoke a reaction of fear in the delirious person.

   (b) *Speech may at times be incoherent* because of slurring and disjointedness.

   (c) *The cycle of sleep and waking may be disrupted* so that the delirious person cannot sleep at night or is drowsy during the day. In some ways, the experiences of a delirious person are like dreams and their behaviour has been described as dreaming while still awake.

   (d) *Activity may be increased or decreased.* Some delirious people become overactive, while others become sluggish. In some cases there may be several switches from overactivity to underactivity during a single day.

Although these criteria treat delirium as a categorical disorder, it is really the severe end of a continuum of clouding of consciousness. Milder states of clouding are probably even more common in the elderly than full-blown delirium, but can be harder to recognise.

RECOGNITION OF DELIRIUM

Although delirium is a temporary state, it is very important to recognise it when it occurs. Delirium often occurs in elderly people when they are suffering from a major physical illness, even if this illness does not directly involve the brain. Indeed, many clinicians recognise that the onset of delirium is often the first sign of a major illness in an elderly person, just as a high temperature or rapid pulse are general signs of illness. Therefore, if delirium is not recognised, a serious illness underlying it may not be identified until too late.

The serious nature of delirium is shown by studies of death rates in delirious patients. A study by Rabins and Folstein (1982) well illustrates the point. They compared a group of hospitalised delirious patients with a group of demented ones. During their hospital admission 23 per cent of the delirious patients died, compared to only 4 per cent of the demented patients. For cognitively intact medical patients the death rate was also 4 per cent. Thus, delirium involves a much greater risk of dying than dementia. Delirious patients also tended to have a higher temperature and more rapid pulse than the demented ones. Again, these are general warning signs of a serious physical illness.

Figures on the frequency of delirium in the elderly are quite varied, but it seems to be quite a common disorder. One geriatrician has reported that as many as 80 per cent of elderly medical patients admitted to a British geriatric unit were suffering from delirium (Bedford, 1959). Most of these patients were admitted directly from their homes and were primarily admitted for general medical rather than psychiatric conditions. Other studies of hospitalised elderly patients have found lower rates of delirium, but the condition is nevertheless quite common. For example, Millar (1981) found that 14 per cent of elderly patients undergoing elective surgery developed delirium in the week following their operation.

Although delirium is not an uncommon problem in the elderly, it is frequently not diagnosed by treating physicians. In one Canadian study of hospitalised medical patients referred for psychiatric consultation, a substantial proportion were found to have delirium. However, in only a third of the cases had the treating physicians realised that delirium was possibly the problem. This was despite the fact that in nearly all cases nurses had recorded distinctive signs of delirium in the person's case notes (Pérez and Silverman, 1984).

In some cases, delirium may not be recognised because it is misdiagnosed as dementia. However, given the very different mortality rates for the two conditions, it is important that they are not confused. Lipowski (1983) has provided a very useful list of features which can be used to differentiate delirium from dementia. These are shown in Table 10.1. Although delirium differs from dementia in many respects, it may be particularly difficult to recognise when superimposed on a pre-existing dementia. However, any sudden worsening or fluctuation in the cognitive function of a demented person would suggest that delirium may be present.

Table 10.1: Features distinguishing delirium from dementia

Feature	Delirium	Dementia
Onset	Rapid, often at night	Usually insidious
Duration	Hours to weeks	Months to years
Course	Fluctuates over 24 hours; worse at night; lucid intervals	Relatively stable
Awareness	Always impaired	Usually normal
Alertness	Reduced or increased; tends to fluctuate	Usually normal
Orientation	Always impaired, at least for time; tendency to mistake unfamiliar for familar place or person	May be intact, little tendency to confabulate
Memory	Recent and immediate impaired; fund of knowledge intact if dementia is absent	Recent and remote impaired; some loss of common knowledge
Thinking	Slow or accelerated; may be dream-like	Poor in abstraction, impoverished
Perception	Often misperceptions, especially visual	Misperceptions often absent
Sleep-wake cycle	Always disrupted; often drowsiness during the day, insomnia at night	Fragmented sleep
Physical illness or drug toxicity	Usually present	Often absent, especially in Alzheimer's disease

Source: adapted from Lipowski (1983)

CAUSES OF DELIRIUM

Delirium can occur at any age, but is much more common in the elderly, particularly those with dementia. As we have seen it is often the first sign of a major physical illness in an elderly person. Although a myriad of factors can lead to delirium, there are a few particularly common causes. These are: toxic effects of drugs, infections, heart disease, and the spreading of cancer throughout the body (Royal College of Physicians, 1981).

The toxic effects of drugs are a particularly common cause of delirium in the elderly. A wide range of drugs, most available only by prescription, can cause delirium, including tranquillisers, sedatives, antidepressants, antiepileptic drugs, some analgesics, and some drugs for the treatment of Parkinson's disease. There are also some drugs which can cause delirium if they are suddenly withdrawn — alcohol and sleeping pills being the most common (Royal College of Physicians, 1981). Perhaps the most notable group of drugs causing delirium in the elderly are those with an anticholinergic action. These drugs disrupt the action of the neurotransmitter acetylcholine which has an important role in cognitive processes such as memory and attention (see Chapter 4). Toxic effects are more likely to arise when elderly people are prescribed many drugs concurrently. If several drugs with anticholinergic effects are being used, the cumulative result can be significant. A large study of prescription practices in the United States found that prescription of multiple anticholinergic drugs for the elderly was not uncommon (Blazer *et al.*, 1983). Between 21 per cent and 32 per cent of nursing home residents were found to be taking two or more drugs with anticholinergic effects. For community-residing elderly people, the figure was between 11 per cent and 13 per cent. A number of nursing home residents were found to be taking five or more anticholinergic drugs! Elderly people are particularly affected by anticholinergics because the supply of acetylcholine to the brain is already decreased with age and becomes markedly decreased in Alzheimer's disease.

Among infections, pneumonia is thought to be a common source of delirium, along with urinary tract infections (Evans, 1982). Sometimes delirium precedes other signs of these infections by a day or more. The manner in which those infections produce delirium is unknown, but some toxins from the infection may pass into the blood-stream and be transported to the brain where they disrupt neurotransmitter function.

Various forms of cardiovascular disease can also cause delirium, usually by affecting the supply of oxygen to the brain since this supply is affected by the state of the heart and blood vessels. The brain is dependent on a supply of oxygen and glucose for its energy requirements and is more sensitive to deprivation than other organs of the body (Bedford, 1959).

The factors which can produce delirium in the elderly are clearly quite varied. However, Evans (1982) has proposed a common mechanism which might explain how delirium can arise through diverse causes. It is known that nerve cells in the brain are constantly active. In fact, information is transmitted from one nerve cell to another by either an increase or decrease in the background level of activity. Evans refers to variation in this background level of activity as *neural noise* and proposes that delirium involves an exacerbation of this noise. If neural noise becomes too great, background activity may be processed as genuine information. Thus, the delirious person sees things that are not really there and has difficulty with memory because irrelevant associations act as a distraction. This increased neural noise is probably due to some disruption to neurotransmitter activity. According to the theory, lack of oxygen to the brain or the presence of toxins may produce this disruption. The theory explains the higher incidence of delirium in the elderly by proposing that their background level of noise is already increased. The blood–brain barrier, acting like a membrane to protect the brain from many chemicals in the blood, may also become impaired with age and allow toxic substances to disrupt brain function.

Given the frequency with which delirium occurs and the increased mortality rates involved, much more attention deserves to be given to this disorder. There is a great need to understand what happens to the brain during delirium, whether there are any long-term effects (such as a greater propensity to become demented), and to evaluate the effectiveness of potential treatments.

11

Assessment of Senile Dementia

INTRODUCTION

Much can be learned about a demented person by clinical examination, informal observation of the person's behaviour and an interview with relatives. However, these activities can be considerably assisted by the use of standard instruments for the assessment of dementia. There are many assessment instruments for dementia which differ in both their purpose and the type of profession which uses them. The simplest assessment devices are the short screening instruments. These give a quick but reliable indication of whether an elderly person has significant cognitive impairment. They do not in themselves provide a full cognitive assessment or allow a diagnosis of dementia to be made, but are a useful indicator of whether further investigation needs to be carried out. More detailed asesssment of cognitive abilities can be made using psychological tests, particularly those concerned with memory and intelligence. The ability to carry out everyday practical tasks such as shopping, bathing and dressing can be assessed by *activities of daily living* scales. These scales are often used by occupational therapists. There are now also standardised procedures for carrying out a formal diagnosis of dementia. These instruments are mainly used in research situations where a standard diagnostic procedure is essential, but are likely to come into more common use in some specialist medical settings. In this chapter, each of these forms of assessment is examined in some detail.

SCREENING FOR DEMENTIA

Screening involves administering a brief test which can select out people who may be demented and therefore require more intensive investigation. These instruments are simple enough to be administered after only brief training and are found quite acceptable by the elderly people to whom they are given. There are many screening instruments available for dementia. Most of these instruments are rather similar in the approach they take and even in the particular questions they use. However, only a few instruments have achieved wide use. Two of the most influential are the Mini-Mental State Examination (MMSE) (see Chapter 9) and the Clifton Assessment Procedures for the Elderly (CAPE).

Mini-Mental State Examination

The MMSE was first described by Folstein, Folstein and McHugh (1975). Since then it has been widely used, but unfortunately several minor variations of the original scale have been introduced. Table 11.1 gives one of the variations, the Diagnostic Interview Schedule version of the MMSE, which will hopefully become the standard. The advantage of this version is that it gives very clear instructions for administering and scoring the MMSE and it has been used in large-scale surveys of elderly people in the community so that there is a great amount of data already available on it.

The MMSE usually takes only around 10 minutes to administer and is rarely found unacceptable or insulting by elderly people. The scoring is reasonably simple. If the number correct on all MMSE questions is added up the greatest possible score is 35. However, in the DIS version the individual being tested is credited with the score either for subtracting 7s from 100 or for spelling WORLD backwards, whichever is the greater. Thus, if a person gets 4 for the subtracting and 5 for WORLD backwards a score of 5 is given for these items. By this method, the total score for the MMSE becomes 30.

Using this version of the MMSE, a person with a score of 24–30 is regarded as having no cognitive impairment, someone with a score of 18–23 is considered to have mild cognitive impairment, and a person scoring 17 or less has severe cognitive impairment. The MMSE has been used in surveys of elderly people living in the community in the United States and Australia. Table 11.2 shows some of the results found. It seems that some degree of cognitive

Table 11.1: The Mini-Mental State Examination (DIS version)

Orientation: (10 points)
    What is the year?
    What is the season?
    What is the day of the week?
    What is the month?
    Can you tell me where we are? (residence or street name required)
    What city/town are we in?
    What state are we in?
    What county are we in? (What are the names of two streets nearby?)
    What floor of the building are we on?
    (WHEN USED IN THE COMMUNITY, THIS QUESTION IS NOT ASKED: SIMPLY SCORE AS CORRECT)
Registration: (3 points)
    I am going to name three objects. After I have said them, I want you to repeat them. Remember what they are because I am going to ask you to name them again in a few minutes. 'Apple . . . Table . . . Penny'.
Attention and calculation: (5 points)
    Can you subtract 7 from 100, and then subtract 7 from the answer you get and keep subtracting 7 until I tell you to stop?
    Now I am going to spell a word forwards and I want you to spell it backwards (in reverse order). The word is WORLD. W-O-R-L-D.
Recall: (3 points)
    Now what were the three objects I asked you to remember?
Language: (9 points)
    What is this called? (Show watch.)
    What is this called? (Show pencil.)
    Now I would like you to repeat a phase after me:
      'No ifs ands or buts.'
    Read the words on this page and then do what it says. (The page says in large letters 'CLOSE YOUR EYES'.)
    Take this paper in your right hand, fold the paper in half using both hands, and put the paper down using your left hand.
    (3 points)
    Pick up the paper and write a short sentence on it for me.
    (Sentence must have a subject and a verb and make sense.)
    Now copy the design that you see printed on the page. (Design is interlocking pentagons. The result must have five-sided figures with intersection forming a four-sided figure.)

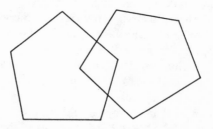

Table 11.2: Cognitive impairment among elderly people living in the community

Age	No impairment (%)	Mild impairment (%)	Severe impariment (%)
	New Haven, United States		
65–74	91	8	1
75–84	77	17	4
85+	59	26	15
	Hobart, Australia		
70+	80	15	5

Source: data from Holzer *et al.* (1984), and Kay *et al.* (1985)

impairment is not uncommon, even amongst elderly people who are living outside nursing homes and hospitals. As would be expected, cognitive impairment becomes increasingly likely with advancing age.

The MMSE is designed to select out people who are likely to be demented. However, because it is strictly a measure of cognitive impairment rather than dementia, low scores can also result because of mental retardation, poor education or learning disability. In spite of its broad nature, the MMSE has been found to be a very good indicator of dementia in the elderly. For example, in one study 97 patients admitted to a general medical ward of a hospital in the United States were screened with the MMSE on admission. Scores of 23 or less were regarded as indicating dementia or delirium. Subsequently, these patients were diagnosed as delirious, demented or normal by a psychiatrist. The MMSE was found to correctly detect 87 per cent of patients suffering from dementia of delirium (Anthony *et al.*, 1982). Amongst patients not suffering from these conditions, it correctly classified them as normal 82 per cent of the time. However, when the MMSE wrongly indicated that dementia might be present, it tended to be with certain sorts of patients. In particular, elderly people with a poor education tended to be erroneously selected as likely cases of dementia. Caution therefore needs to be exercised when the MMSE is used as a screening instrument for such people.

Despite its brevity, scores on the MMSE have been found to relate well to performance on lengthy intelligence tests such as the Wechsler Adult Intelligence Scale (discussed more fully below). The MMSE can be regarded as a crude test of general intelligence for people scoring below the population average. For people of average or above average intelligence, however, the MMSE is of little use because they will all get perfect or near perfect scores.

Clifton Assessment Procedures for the Elderly (CAPE)

The CAPE (Pattie and Gilleard, 1979) is made up of two parts organised as shown in Figure 11.1. The first part is the Cognitive Assessment Scale which is similar in purpose to the MMSE. The Cognitive Assessment Scale itself has three components: an information/orientation scale with questions like 'What day is it?' and 'Who is the Prime Minister?'; a mental ability scale with tasks like counting from 1 to 20 and writing one's name; and a psychomotor scale which involves tracing the correct path through a maze.

The second part of the CAPE, the Behaviour Rating Scale, is filled out by a nurse or someone very familiar with the elderly person's behaviour. Ratings are made for specific behaviours in the areas of physical disability, apathy, communication difficulties, and social disturbance. For example, in the physical disability section, the rater has to say whether the elderly person bathes or dresses with no assistance (0 points), some assistance (1 point) or maximum assistance (2 points). Similarly, there is a rating of whether the person is in bed during the day; never (0 points), sometimes (1 point) or almost always (2 points). Altogether, there are six ratings made in the section on physical disability to give a maximum score of 12 points. A similar approach is adopted in the sections dealing with apathy, communication difficulties and social disturbance.

The CAPE has been used with elderly people largely in institutional settings. Here it is used to grade people according to the type and severity of their disabilities. Patients hospitalised for organic disorders like dementia have been found to do worse on both the Cognitive Assessment Scale and the Behaviour Rating Scale than patients with psychiatric disorders like depression and schizophrenia. Furthermore, patients with poor scores on the CAPE were found to be less likely to be discharged from hospital and return home (Pattie and Gilleard, 1975).

More recently, a briefer *Survey* version of the CAPE has been developed (Pattie, 1981). This version is more useful in screening. It consists of the information/orientation component of the Cognitive Assessment Scale and the physical-disability component of the Behaviour Rating Scale. The Survey version of the CAPE was developed because it was found that scores on all sections of the CAPE are highly related. Thus, people with poor scores on one test of the Cognitive Assessment Scale tended to have poor scores on the other tests, and similarly with the Behaviour Rating Scale. Because all components of the CAPE appear to be assessing the same

Figure 11.1: Organisation of the Clifton Assessment Procedures for the Elderly (CAPE)

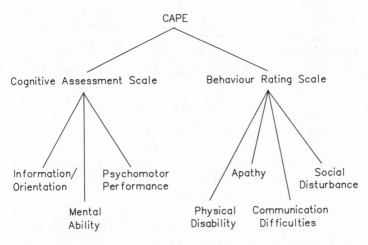

dimension of dependency, it is possible to shorten the assessment by using only the information/orientation and physical disability components. These two components can be pooled to give an overall assessment of dependency by subtracting the physical disability score from the information/orientation score. Someone with no errors on information/orientation and no rated physical disability would get the best score of +12, while at the other extreme, a person with errors on all the information/orientation questions and the maximum ratings for physical disability would score −12. As might be expected dependency scores are closely related to the degree of care an elderly person is receiving. People living in the community average 9.4, while geriatric and psychogeriatric patients average 0.5 and 0.4 respectively. When elderly people with different dependency scores were followed up over a two-year period, those with greater dependency were more likely to die during the period.

While the Survey version of the CAPE clearly distinguishes *groups* of people according to the level of care they are receiving, it may not be sufficiently accurate for use in assigning *individual* patients to types of care (McPherson *et al.*, 1985). It needs to be remembered that this is a screening instrument and does not provide a full assessment of an elderly person's competencies and limitations. Rather, screening instruments simply indicate the need for further investigation to be carried out.

93

PSYCHOLOGICAL TESTING IN DEMENTIA

Two aspects of mental ability invariably affected in dementia are intelligence and memory, so it is natural that psychological tests for these attributes should be widely used with demented patients. Undoubtedly the most widely used adult tests for these abilities are the Wechsler Adult Intelligence Scale and the Wechsler Memory Scale.

Wechsler Adult Intelligence Scale

The Wechsler Adult Intelligence Scale (WAIS) was first published in 1955 but was revised in 1981. The updated version is referred to as the WAIS-R. The WAIS-R is divided into two parts: the Verbal Scale which measures aspects of intelligence involving language, and the Performance Scale which measures non-verbal problem-solving skills. These two scales are each made up of a series of tests as shown in Table 11.3. Using the WAIS-R it is possible to get an overall IQ score, Verbal and Performance IQ scores, as well as scores on all the individual tests.

The WAIS-R has been given to a large number of people representative of the United States population. Scores on the test are derived by comparing the individual being tested with this normative group. Scores are expressed as IQs, where 100 means that a person performs at the average for his or her age group. The meaning of various other IQ scores is shown in Table 11.4.

When the WAIS-R was given to the normative sample, it was found that elderly people tend to do more poorly than young and middle-aged adults. Thus an IQ of 100 for a 40-year-old does not mean exactly the same level of performance as an IQ of 100 for a 70-year-old. Although both are average for their age, the average performance of 70-year-olds is worse than that of 40-year-olds.

A major limitation of WAIS-R for use with elderly people is that no normative data were gathered on people aged 75 or over, yet it is in this age group that dementia is most common. Also, data on countries besides the United States are not available, so that other English-speaking countries must rely on American data which may not be strictly applicable. Nevertheless, the WAIS-R can be a very useful tool in the investigation of dementia.

Of the greatest interest in dementia is not the overall IQ score, but the patterning of test scores in terms of relative strengths and

Table 11.3: Tests making up the Wechsler Adult Intelligence Scale-Revised (WAIS-R)

Verbal scale	What it involves
Information	Answering general knowledge questions
Digit span	Holding digits in memory for a few seconds
Vocabulary	Defining the meanings of words
Arithmetic	Solving mental arithmetic problems
Comprehension	Knowing the reasons for social conventions
Similarities	Explaining the way in which two things are alike
Performance scale	
Picture completion	Finding the missing parts of incomplete pictures
Picture arrangement	Ordering a series of cartoon pictures to make a story
Block design	Making abstract patterns out of blocks
Object assembly	Solving jigsaw puzzles
Digit symbol	Rapidly writing abstract symbols beneath numbers which they go with

Table 11.4: Interpretation of IQ Scores on the WAIS-R

IQ	Description	Percentage of population receiving such scores
130+	Very superior	2
120–129	Superior	7
110–109	High average	16
90–109	Average	50
80–89	Low average	16
70–79	Borderline	7
–69	Mentally retarded	2

weaknesses. For example, it has been found repeatedly that the Performance IQ tends to be lower in dementia than the Verbal IQ (Inglis, 1958; Alexander, 1973). Nevertheless, in a minority of dementia cases the Performance IQ will still be higher, and in many normal elderly people the Performance IQ will be lower, so this difference cannot be regarded as a completely reliable diagnostic sign. Even more specific patterning of WAIS test scores in dementia has been reported by Fuld (1983). She has found that Alzheimer's disease patients often have a pattern of strengths and weaknesses different from that seen in other types of dementia or in normal ageing. This pattern involves the Information, Vocabulary, Similarities, Digit Span, Digit Symbol, Block Design and Object Assembly tests.

Least impairment is found on the Information and Vocabulary tests, somewhat more on Similarities and Digit Span, most on Digit Symbol and Block Design, with Object Assembly occupying an intermediate position somewhere between the best and worst tests. Note that performance is best on tests which assess information acquired in the past, while worst performance is on tests involving novel situations. Fuld claims that around 50 per cent of Alzheimer's disease patients who can be tested on the WAIS (some are too impaired to be tested at all) show this pattern, whereas less than 1 per cent of normal elderly people show it.

Estimating pre-morbid intelligence

When testing intelligence in demented people, the interest is often not so much in their current score as in estimating how much they have declined. Thus, a demented person of superior intelligence may decline to average intelligence and still do better than many normal people. By contrast, a person who has always been of low intelligence may be mistakenly regarded as demented, even though they have declined very little. Tests like the WAIS-R give a measure of a person's present state of intelligence, but what is also needed is an estimate of intelligence earlier in life. In some rare instances, a test of intelligence may have been given earlier in life, but in most cases an indirect approach has to be used to estimate premorbid intelligence.

Three approaches have been tried with varying success. The simplest is to use social class indicators like occupation, education and race to estimate premorbid IQ. It is known that these attributes are related to a person's intelligence, so they can be used to predict it. Wilson, Rosenbaum and Brown (1979) have developed a statistical formula for use in the United States based on this principle. This formula is:

Estimated IQ = 0.17 × age −1.53 × sex −11.33 × race + 2.97 × education + 1.01 × occupation + 74.05

In this formula, male = 1, female = 2, white = 1, non-white = 2, education is measured in years of schooling, and occupation is measured on an 11-point scale where, for example, farm labourers get 0, clerical sales and kindred workers get 7, and students get 10. Thus, a 60-year-old white female clerical worker with 10 years of education would have the following estimated IQ:

Estimated IQ $= 0.17 \times 60 -1.53 \times 2 -11.33 \times 1 + 2.97 \times 10 + 1.01 \times 7 + 74.05 = 107$

If this woman had a measured IQ of 70 on the WAIS-R we would expect that she had suffered some intellectual decline. Unfortunately, this approach gives only a very crude estimate and is not accurate enough to establish reliably the premorbid IQs of individual patients. It is probably also inappropriate for use outside the United States because of the different educational systems and racial compositions in other countries.

An alternative approach is to use abilities which hold up well in dementia to estimate premorbid intelligence. One very early approach of this sort was to use the WAIS Vocabulary score because it has been found to be less affected in dementia than the other WAIS tests. However, Vocabulary is not ideal in this regard because it does show some decline in dementia (Nelson and McKenna, 1975) and so underestimates a demented person's premorbid intelligence.

Undoubtedly the most successful approach to date towards estimating premorbid intelligence is the use of word reading tests. Nelson and McKenna (1975) first made the interesting observation that the ability to read lists of words is remarkably well preserved in dementia. Because word reading ability is highly related to IQ in adults, it can be used as an estimator of premorbid IQ. The initial work on word reading in dementia used the Schonell Graded Word Reading Test which was originally devised for measuring reading skill in children. It consists of 100 words graded in difficulty from very easy to quite hard. These words are shown in Table 11.5. Testing starts with the easiest words and continues until ten errors are made in a row. The number of words read correctly can be used to predict WAIS IQ using the following formula:

Predicted IQ $= 44.1 + 0.71 \times$ Schonell score

Thus, a person reading 90 of the Schonell words correctly would be predicted to have an IQ of: $44.1 + 0.71 \times 90 = 108$. This predicted IQ can then be compared to the actually obtained IQ to see whether intellectual decline has occurred.

A limitation of the Schonell Graded Word Reading Test is that it does not discriminate amongst very intelligent people because they usually get all 100 words correct. A list of more difficult words is needed. Recognition of this problem led Nelson and O'Connell (1978) to develop a new reading test variously known as the *New*

Table 11.5: Words used in the Schonell Graded Word Reading Test

tree	little	milk	egg	book
school	sit	frog	playing	bun
flower	road	clock	train	light
picture	think	summer	people	something
dream	downstairs	biscuit	shepherd	thirsty
crowd	sandwich	beginning	postage	island
saucer	angel	ceiling	appeared	gnome
canary	attractive	imagine	nephew	gradually
smoulder	applaud	disposal	nourished	diseased
university	orchestra	knowledge	audience	situated
physics	campaign	choir	intercede	fascinate
forfeit	siege	recent	plausible	prophecy
colonel	soloist	systematic	slovenly	classification
genuine	institution	pivot	conscience	heroic
pneumonia	preliminary	antique	susceptible	enigma
oblivion	scintillate	satirical	sabre	beguile
terrestrial	belligerent	adamant	sepulchre	statistics
miscellaneous	procrastinate	tyrannical	evangelical	grotesque
ineradicable	judicature	preferential	homonym	fictitious
rescind	metamorphosis	somnambulist	bibliography	idiosyncrasy

Source: Schonell and Schonell (1952)

Adult Reading Test, *Nelson Adult Reading Test* and *National Adult Reading Test*. Fortunately, the various names all yield the same acronym: NART. The NART consists of 50 difficult words which were selected because they are irregular in spelling and would not be read correctly by someone unfamiliar with them. Examples of such words are CELLIST, SIMILE and NAIVE. Several studies have now shown that the Schonell Graded Word Reading Test and the NART provide quite good estimations of a demented person's premorbid ability (Ruddell and Bradshaw, 1982; Hart, Smith and Swash, 1986). However, caution still needs to be exercised in individual cases because general intelligence is being estimated on the basis of only one skill. Some people (for example those with a specific reading disability) may be very poor at reading, yet quite intelligent in other respects. For them, an estimate of premorbid intelligence on the basis of a word reading test could give quite a misleading picture.

Table 11.6: Tests making up the Wechsler Memory Scale

Test	What it involves
Personal and current information	Giving information about oneself and people in the news
Orientation	Knowing the date and place
Mental control	Counting backwards, repeating the alphabet, and counting by 3s
Logical memory	Recalling the ideas in two passages
Memory span	Holding digits in memory for a few seconds
Visual reproduction	Drawing simple geometric figures from memory
Associate learning	Learning to associate pairs of words together, so that when one is given by the tester the other can be recalled

Wechsler Memory Scale

The Wechsler Memory Scale has been widely used to assess memory function in demented people. This test is quite old, being first published in 1945 and not revised since (Wechsler and Stone, 1945). The Wechsler Memory Scale consists of seven tests covering different aspects of memory. These are shown in Table 11.6. As well as scores on the individual tests, the Wechsler Memory Scale yields an overall *memory quotient* which is interpreted much like an IQ score. Like the WAIS-R, the Wechsler Memory Scale has been given to a normative group to which an individual's score can be compared. However, a major limitation is that this normative group was tested over 40 years ago and even then was not representative of the United States population. Furthermore, the normative group did not include anyone over age 50, thereby totally excluding the age group at risk for dementia. There are, however, more recent normative data for the Wechsler Memory Scale using an Australian sample, with people up to age 69 included (Ivison, 1977). This comparison group is probably better than Wechsler's original normative group.

It is apparent from comparing the contents of the Wechsler Memory Scale with those of the WAIS-R, that there is some overlap in the skills required in each. In fact, it has been found that scores on the WAIS relate quite well to those on the Wechsler Memory Scale. Thus, intelligence and memory, as measured in these scales, are not independent attributes of a person.

Probably the major limitation of the Wechsler Memory Scale is its age. At the time it was devised there was very little understanding of either normal memory processes or memory disorders. In the light of contemporary knowledge, it appears very dated in its content. In more recent years there has been growing interest in tests of memory which can specifically assess particular underlying memory functions. One such task is the Buschke Selective Reminding Task.

Buschke Selective Reminding Task

This task does not constitute a memory test in the same sense as the Wechsler Memory Scale. Rather, it is an approach towards measuring various memory processes which can be quite useful in the assessment of dementia.

The selective reminding task (Buschke and Fuld, 1974) involves learning a list of words. Any list of words can be used, but they should be homogeneous for difficulty and the length of the list should be such as to provide a reasonable challenge for the person being tested. Lists of ten to twelve words are generally suitable for demented patients. The words on the list are read out at the rate of one every 2 seconds. At the end of the list, the person being tested has to recall as many words as possible in any order they wish. On the next trial the list is presented again omitting any words recalled correctly on the previous trial. This procedure can be repeated for any number of trials, but five to ten are usually optimal. The task is referred to as *selective reminding* because there is reminding only of those words missed on the previous trial.

Table 11.7 shows an example of how a ten-word list might be used in a selective reminding task. On the first trial, all ten words are presented, but only four of these are correctly recalled. On the second trial, only the six words not recalled on the previous trial are presented. After this presentation, five words are recalled, two of which were reminded (*kangaroo* and *fox*) and three of which were not (*deer, moose* and *cow*). The selective reminding process then continues for three more trials, after which all the words are recalled correctly.

The advantage of using the selective reminding procedure is that it allows separate measures to be made of long-term storage, long-term retrieval and short-term recall (compare Chapter 5). When a word is correctly recalled on a particular trial there is no reminding of it on the next trial. If it can be recalled without reminding then

Table 11.7: Example of the Selective Reminding Task

TRIAL 1		TRIAL 2		TRIAL 3	
Presented	*Recalled*	*Presented*	*Recalled*	*Presented*	*Recalled*
deer	deer		deer		deer
kangaroo		kangaroo	kangaroo		kangaroo
antelope		antelope		antelope	
elephant		elephant		elephant	elephant
fox		fox	fox		
llama		llama		llama	
tiger		tiger		tiger	
bear	bear			bear	bear
moose	moose		moose		moose
cow	cow		cow		

TRIAL 4		TRIAL 5	
Presented	*Recalled*	*Presented*	*Recalled*
	deer		deer
	kangaroo		kangaroo
antelope	antelope		antelope
	elephant		elephant
fox	fox		fox
llama		llama	llama
tiger	tiger		tiger
	bear		bear
	moose		moose
cow	cow		cow

it is in long-term storage. Thus, in Table 11.7, *deer* was recalled correctly on trial 2 without reminding. Therefore, we would conclude that it had been placed in long-term storage on trial 1 when it was first recalled. If, however, a word is recalled when there is reminding, but not on the next trial without reminding, short-term recall must have been used. For example, in Table 11.7 *bear* was recalled after the word was presented on trial 1, but not on the second trial without reminding. Therefore, *bear* was remembered by short-term recall on trial 1.

Sometimes a word gets into long-term storage, but is later not recalled correctly. This is an example of retrieval failure. For example, *cow* was recalled on trial 1 after the word was presented. It was also recalled on trial 2 even though not presented on this trial. Therefore, it must have been placed in long-term storage on trial 1. However, on trial 3, it was not recalled, indicating a failure to retrieve it from long-term storage. By counting up examples of long-term storage, short-term recall and long-term retrieval, it is possible to get separate estimates of these memory processes and to discover specifically why memory is poor.

Table 11.8: Example of the use of the Selective Reminding Task to evaluate a new drug treatment

Day number	Activity
1	Selective Reminding Task 1
2–11	No treatment
13	Selective Reminding Task 2
14–23	Placebo treatment
24	Selective Reminding Task 3
25–34	Drug treatment
35	Selective Reminding Task 4
36–45	Placebo treatment
46	Selective Reminding Task 5

The selective reminding task is most useful in evaluating memory deterioration or improvement in dementia. By using a large pool of homogeneous words (a useful word pool is provided by Kraemer *et al.*, 1983), it is possible to produce numerous different versions of the selective reminding task, each of similar difficulty. Thus, in evaluating whether a new drug treatment is improving memory in a demented person, different versions of the test can be given at various times to monitor whether improvement is occurring. Such a use is illustrated in Table 11.8. Traditional memory tests like the Wechsler Memory Scale are not so useful in such situations. Patients will improve as they repeat the test simply because they are becoming more practised on the particular tasks being used.

Kendrick Battery for the Detection of Dementia

None of the psychological tests described above is specifically designed for use with demented people. Rather, they are tests of cognitive function which are useful in a wide range of situations. By contrast, there is a psychological test, the *Kendrick Battery for the Detection of Dementia in the Elderly* (Gibson and Kendrick, 1979), which is specifically designed to assess the cognitive deficits typical of dementia.

The Kendrick Battery consists of two tests: the Object Learning Test and the Digit Copying Test. These are designed to assess cognitive abilities which are prone to decline with age, such as learning and mental speed. The Object Learning Test involves showing the elderly person large cards with pictures on them. For example, the first card has pictures of a cat, bed, watch, key, banana, horse, spectacles, newspaper, spoon and jug. This card is shown for 30 seconds and then the elderly person must recall as many objects on the card as they can in any order. Three more cards are shown, each with more objects to remember than the last. The hardest card has 25 objects and is shown for 75 seconds. The number of objects remembered over all four cards is simply totalled to give a measure of learning.

The Digit Copying Test consists of a page of 100 digits. The elderly person has to copy the digits by writing them underneath the ones on the page as fast as possible. Two minutes are allowed for this task, and the person's score is the number of digits copied in this time.

The Kendrick Battery is designed to be given on two occasions wherever possible so as to demonstrate that decline is occurring. With the Digit Copying Test, it is possible to do it a second time without practice effects creating problems. However, practice is a problem with a memory test like the Object Learning Test, so two equivalent versions of this test have been devised.

The Kendrick Battery has been found to be quite successful at differentiating clear cases of dementia from clearly normal people (Kendrick, Gibson and Moyes, 1979). However, a major use of psychological tests is to assist where the diagnosis of dementia is uncertain. For example, mild dementia can be difficult to assess in people of high or low premorbid intelligence, yet the Kendrick Battery provides measures of current cognitive function which do not take into account premorbid skills.

Computerised testing

An approach that is beginning to claim attention is the use of computers to assess cognitive function in the elderly. Because of the availability of ever cheaper microcomputers, it is natural to consider the degree to which labour-intensive psychological testing can be automated. In fact, a number of pilot projects have already been carried out demonstrating the acceptability of computerised testing to elderly people (Carr et al., 1982; Ogden et al., 1984).

There are particular problems in using computers to test the elderly: computers are generally unfamiliar to elderly people and they often have problems with vision, hearing, or movement which make it difficult for them to respond appropriately. Much of the pilot work with computerised testing has been concerned with producing large legible screen displays and providing an easy response mode, such as pressing large buttons.

Although computerised testing will undoubtedly be useful in some situations, it is unlikely to replace the human tester. Much of the effort in testing the elderly is in gaining cooperation and making the person feel at ease, and these are human skills which are difficult to transfer to a computer. Most existing tests (such as the Wechsler scales) have been designed for human administration and scoring and would be difficult or impossible to transfer to a computer. For example, the Block Design test of the WAIS-R requires the person to pick up, rotate and place blocks in appropriate ways. People find the actual manipulation of the blocks easy and can concentrate on the more difficult problem of arranging them correctly according to the pattern. Such a test could be transferred to a computer screen, but the programming effort involved would be considerable and the person being tested would require detailed and complicated instruction on how to manipulate the blocks on the screen.

Although there are many aspects of testing that humans do better than computers, computers do have advantages in some areas. Currently used tests are designed to make use of the human tester's strengths and it would make little sense to adapt these tests for computerised presentation. A better approach is to design new tests for the computer which make use of its particular strengths in relation to human testers. For example, most human-administered tests yield a score by counting the number of correct responses. It is easy for humans to count number correct, but this is only one of several possible measures of performance. Response times and type of error are others. Good performance involves faster responses, but few tests use this measure because humans are poor at accurately recording reponse times to individual questions. For computers, however, measurement of response time is easily programmed. Similarly, the type of errors a person makes can sometimes tell us as much as the actual number of errors made, but scoring of type of error is time-consuming for human testers.

Another area where computers have an advantage is in tailoring the difficulty of questions to suit the ability of the person being tested. The cognitive abilities of elderly people encompass an enormous range. Questions which are difficult and threatening to one person may be insultingly easy to another. Often tests involve presenting questions in order of difficulty, starting with the easiest and stopping after a certain number of errors. However, for a bright person the easy items at the beginning of the test can be tedious.

Computers can, in principle, tailor the questions being asked to suit the individual by selecting additional questions on the basis of performance on already completed questions. Human testers, by contrast, find it difficult to work through a list of questions in any sort of complex order.

The development of computerised tests for the elderly is still in its early stages. Judgement on the usefulness of this approach must await the final development of tests specifically designed to use the computer's strengths, yet acceptable to elderly users.

ASSESSING SKILLS OF DAILY LIVING

There are certain activities which must be carried out in daily life to achieve independent living. These include dressing, bathing, toileting, feeding and moving about one's home. Anyone who is unable to perform some of these essential activities will require assistance from others. The most dependent cases will require institutional care.

Many scales have been developed to measure everyday living skills. These scales are of use not only with the demented, but also with elderly people having other health problems such as strokes and fractured hips. Such assessments can be used to guide rehabilitation programmes and can assist in decisions about the most appropriate placement for an elderly person. For example, when elderly people admitted to hospital with stroke are due for discharge, it is necessary to know whether they can return home and live independently, require some assistance at home, or are so disabled that they need nursing home care.

Several different approaches to the assessment of daily living skills have been tried. The most commonly used is observation of the elderly person's performance in a hospital ward. The earliest scale of daily living skills, developed by Katz and his colleagues (1963), uses this approach. This scale is called the Index of Independence in Activities of Daily Living, or Index of ADL for short. This instrument was originally developed on the basis of observations of patients with fracture of the hip. However, it has since been applied to elderly people with a wide range of health problems, including dementia. The Index of ADL is shown in Tables 11.9 and 11.10. To use this instrument, an observer fills out the evaluation form shown in Table 11.10. This requires observation of skills in bathing, dressing, toileting, transferring in and out of bed

Table 11.9: Evaluation form for the Index of ADL

For each area of functioning listed below, check description that applies. (The word 'assistance' means supervision, direction, or personal assistance.)

Bathing: either sponge bath; tub bath, or shower.

☐	☐	☐
Receives no assistance (gets in and out of tub by self if tub is usual means of bathing)	Receives assistance in bathing only one part of the body (such as back or a leg)	Receives assistance in bathing more than one part of the body (or not bathed)

Dressing: gets clothes from closets and drawers — including underclothes, outer garments and using fasteners (including braces if worn)

☐	☐	☐
Gets clothes and gets completely dressed without assistance	Gets clothes and gets completely dressed without assistance except for assistance in tying shoes	Receives assistance in getting clothes or in getting dressed, or stays partly or completely undressed

Toileting: going to the 'toilet room' for bowel and urine elimination; cleaning self after elimination, and arranging clothes

☐	☐	☐
Goes to 'toilet room', cleans self, and arranges clothes without assistance (may use object for support such as cane, walker, or wheelchair and may manage night bedpan or commode, emptying same in morning)	Receives assistance in going to 'toilet room' or in cleansing self or in arranging clothes after elimination or in use of night bedpan or commode	Doesn't go to room termed 'toilet' for the elimination process

Transfer

☐	☐	☐
Moves in and out of bed as well as in and out of chair without assistance (may be using object for support such as cane or walker)	Moves in and out of bed or chair with assistance	Doesn't get out of bed

Continence

☐	☐	☐
Controls urination and bowel movement completely by self	Has occasional 'accidents'	Supervision helps keep urine or bowel control; catheter is used, or is incontinent

Feeding

☐	☐	☐
Feeds self without assistance	Feeds self except for getting assistance in cutting meat or buttering bread	Receives assistance in feeding or is fed partly or completely by using tubes or intravenous fluids

Source: Katz *et al.* (1963)

106

Table 11.10: Index of Independence in Activities of Daily Living

The Index of Independence in Activities of Daily Living is based on an evaluation of the functional independence or dependence of patients in bathing, dressing, going to toilet, transferring, continence, and feeding. Specific definitions of functional independence and dependence appear below the index.

A: Independent in feeding, continence, transferring, going to toilet, dressing, and bathing.

B: Independent in all but one of these functions.

C: Independent in all but bathing and one additional function.

D: Independent in all but bathing, dressing, and one additional function.

E: Independent in all but bathing, dressing, going to toilet, and one additional functional.

F: Independent in all but bathing, dressing, going to toilet, transferring, and one additional function.

G: Dependent in all six functions.

Other: Dependent in at least two functions, but not classifiable as C, D, E, or F.

Independence means without supervision, direction, or active personal assistance, except as specifically noted below. This is based on actual status and not on ability. A patient who refuses to perform a function is considered as not performing the function, even though he is deemed able.

Bathing (sponge, shower, or tub)
Independent: assistance only in bathing a single part (as back or disabled extremity) or bathes self completely

Dependent: assistance in bathing more than one part of the body; assistance in getting in or out of tub or does not bathe self

Dressing
Independent: gets clothes from closets and drawers; puts on clothes, outer garments, braces; manages fasteners; act of tying shoes is excluded

Dependent: does not dress self or remains partly undressed

Going to toilet
Independent: gets to toilet: gets on and off toilet; arranges clothes; cleans organs of excretion (may manage own bedpan used at night only and may or may not be using mechanical supports

Dependent: uses bedpan or commode or receives assistance in getting to and using toilet

Transfer
Independent: moves in and out of bed independently and moves in and out of chair independently (may or may not be using mechanical supports)

Dependent: assistance in moving in or out of bed and/or chair; does not perform one or more transfers

Continence
Independent: urination and defaecation entirely self-controlled

Dependent: partial or total incontinence in urination or defaection; partial or total control by enemas, catheters, or regulated use of urinals and/or bedpans

Feeding
Independent: gets food from plate or its equivalent into mouth (precutting of meat and preparation of food, as buttering bread, are excluded from evaluation)

Dependent: assistance in act of feeding, (see above); does not eat at all or parenteral feeding

Source: Katz *et al.* (1963)

or a chair, continence and feeding. Ratings of performance at these skills are then used to assess whether the person is dependent or independent at each activity using the definitions given at the top of Table 11.10. The elderly person is then assigned to one of the levels of independence shown in the lower half of Table 11.10. Using this index, a person assessed at level A would be able to live independently, a person at levels B or C would need assistance at some times, while a person at lower levels would require assistance more frequently.

Sometimes the observation time necessary to use scales like the Index of ADL is not possible. For example, it might be necessary to assess daily living skills during a short interview or in someone who is temporarily bedridden. An alternative approach is to ask the elderly person to perform various tasks in an actual test situation. This approach is used in the Performance Test of Activities of Daily Living (PADL) (Kuriansky and Gurland, 1976). The PADL consists of the sixteen tasks shown in Table 11.11. Notice that all the tasks require the use of portable props. As each of these tasks involves several component skills, points are given for each component not successfully managed. For example, for combing hair, points are given for not being able to (a) take the comb in hand, (b) grasp the comb properly, (c) bring the comb to the hair, and (d) make combing motions. The whole test generally takes only about 20 minutes to complete.

The performance approach to assessing daily living skills has some advantage over the observational approach in that it tests what the elderly person *can* do rather than what they *do* do. For example, a demented person may not feed herself through apathy, yet be quite capable of doing so when encouraged. Thus the PADL gets more directly at physical incapacity independent of any lack of motivation.

STANDARDISED PSYCHIATRIC EXAMINATIONS

To be diagnosed as demented, a person is examined by a psychiatrist or other specialist who decides whether certain symptoms are present. If the symptoms conform to the pattern specified in some diagnostic criteria for dementia (see Chapter 1), then a diagnosis of the disorder is made. By using a particular set of diagnostic criteria it is possible to ensure, to a certain degree, that there is diagnostic consistency from one diagnostician to another and by the same person from occasion to occasion. However, even when using a

Table 11.11: Tasks used in the Performance Test of Activities of Daily Living

Task Requests	Props to be used
1. Drink from a cup	Cup
2. Use a tissue to wipe nose	Tissue Box
3. Comb hair	Comb
4. File nails	Nail file
5. Shave	Shaver
6. Lift food onto spoon and to mouth	Spoon with candy on it
7. Turn tap on and off	Tap
8. Turn light switch on and off	Light switch
9. Put on and remove a jacket with buttons	Jacket
10. Put on and remove a slipper	Slipper
11. Brush teeth, including removing false ones	Toothbrush
12. Make a phone call	Telephone
13. Sign name	Paper and pen
14. Turn key in lock	Keyhole and key
15. Tell time	Clock
16. Stand up and walk a few steps and sit back down	

Source: Kuriansky and Gurland (1976)

particular set of criteria there will still be disagreement about the correct diagnosis in a substantial percentage of cases. These disagreements arise because diagnosticians ask different questions during an examination and interpret the diagnostic criteria somewhat differently.

One way of reducing such disagreements is to use a standard procedure for the examination and to apply the diagnostic criteria to the resulting information using a computer program. In recent years, several standard psychiatric examinations have been devised to achieve greater diagnostic agreement. Some of these are specifically designed for use with elderly people and so incorporate questions which allow a diagnosis of dementia to be made. Three such standardised examinations are described in this section: the Geriatric Mental State Schedule (GMS), the Comprehensive Assessment and Referral Evaluation (CARE), and the Cambridge Mental Disorders of the Elderly Examination (CAMDEX).

Geriatric Mental State Schedule (GMS)

The GMS (Copeland *et al.*, 1976) was developed out of earlier standardised interviews meant for younger adults. These earlier interviews proved to be unsuitable for the elderly in a number of ways, not least of which was that they did not cover conditions like dementia which are rare in younger age groups.

In the GMS, patients are questioned about how they have been feeling in the month prior to interview. In addition there are questions to assess the person's current cognitive abilities. The interviewer uses the patient's responses to rate the severity of over 500 different symptoms. Table 11.12 gives two brief excerpts from the GMS, the first dealing with cognitive impairment and the second covering certain symptoms of depression. These excerpts give a general idea of the types of questions asked and how ratings are carried out on the basis of the elderly person's responses. Rating these symptoms requires special training. It is recommended that a person learn how to use the GMS by undertaking 20 joint interviews with an instructor, with each interview being followed by a discussion of any discrepancies in ratings. However, an advantage of a standardised interview like the GMS is that non-psychiatrists can be trained to carry out a psychiatric examination. The GMS takes around 30 or 40 minutes to administer in most cases, although longer interviews are sometimes necessary.

Once the ratings are made by the interviewer they can be analysed by a set of rules called AGECAT which are written in the form of a computer program. The procedure used by AGECAT to arrive at a diagnosis is quite complex, but basically it involves sorting the symptoms ratings into eight broad clusters or syndromes. The scores on these clusters are used to arrive at a main diagnosis and, where appropriate, an alternative diagnosis. The advantage of using AGECAT is that once the symptom ratings are completed the same diagnosis will always result, whereas different psychiatrists making a diagnosis on the basis of the same information will not always agree. The disadvantage is that AGECAT requires computer processing and cannot produce an immediate diagnosis if one is required.

Several studies have compared AGECAT diagnoses with those of experienced psychiatrists, and have shown high levels of agreement, particularly for dementia and depression. In fact, AGECAT agrees with psychiatrists' diagnoses to much the same extent as psychiatrists agree with each other in their diagnostic decisions.

At present, the GMS is based completely on a psychiatric examination of the elderly person. However, psychiatrists generally have other sources of information available to them which can improve their diagnoses, such as a history of any problems obtained from a relative and a physical examination. The GMS is currently being updated to incorporate these sources of information, which should eventually produce even better results.

Comprehensive Assessment and Referral Evaluation (CARE)

The CARE was based on the GMS but with the addition of many new items covering medical and social as well as psychiatric problems. Originally, the CARE contained 1500 items and took an average of 1½ hours to administer. A month of training was considered necessary before someone could properly carry out this long interview. Obviously, a detailed and lengthy interview of this sort would not find widespread use, so shorter versions of the CARE were produced (Gurland and Wilder, 1984). Here we describe one of those versions, the SHORT-CARE, which is made up of 143 items dealing with dementia, depression and disability (Gurland *et al.*, 1984). The SHORT-CARE takes a little over half an hour to administer and non-psychiatrists can be trained in its use.

The SHORT-CARE can diagnose dementia and depression in two ways. The first is to apply a set of complex diagnostic criteria to the interview items to arrive at diagnoses of *pervasive dementia* and *pervasive depression* (Gurland *et al.*, 1984). In some cases, these diagnoses can be more accurate than those made by psychiatrists using the traditional clinical approach. For example, when demented people are followed up over a year, they would be expected to deteriorate, with many dying or entering institutional care. If they do not deteriorate, the original diagnosis may have been inappropriate. In one study, the diagnosis of pervasive dementia using the SHORT-CARE items was found to be better at predicting this deterioration than psychiatrists' diagnoses. Some of the people diagnosed as demented by psychiatrists had not deteriorated at follow-up.

The second method of diagnosis is simpler and involves the use of *diagnostic scales*. These scales simply involve adding up symptoms of dementia and depression (Golden, Teresi and Gurland, 1983). The diagnostic scale for dementia contains seventeen symptoms such as *doesn't know address, doesn't know year, another person does shopping*, and *difficulty dressing self*. Similarly, there are eighteen symptoms of depression, including *feels lonely, worries, feels future is bleak* and *awakes early or tired*. Best results were obtained when both these diagnostic scales were used together

111

Table 11.12: Some excerpts from the Geriatric Mental State Schedule (Version 6)

Excerpt 1

1. I WOULD LIKE YOU TO REMEMBER MY NAME. MY NAME IS ____ CAN YOU REPEAT THAT? (Reiterate name until correctly repeated.)
    Correctly repeated
    Cannot repeat interviewer's name correctly after three or less repetitions. Minor mispronunciations are allowed
    No answer, no codable reply

2. PLEASE SPELL YOUR LAST NAME (FOR ME). AND YOUR FIRST NAME?
    If patient says he does not now, press gently once or twice for a reply saying: COULD YOU PLEASE TRY TO TELL ME?
    Correctly spelled
    Cannot give both names correctly. One minor spelling error allowed
    No answer, no codable reply

3. WHAT YEAR WERE YOU BORN?
    Year _____
    Does not know
    No answer, no codable reply

4. HOW OLD ARE YOU?
    Age in years _____
    Does not know
    No answer, no codable reply

5. WHAT DAY OF THE WEEK IS IT TODAY?
    Day _____
    Does not know
    No answer, no codable reply

6. WHAT MONTH IS IT?
    Month _____
    Does not know
    No answer, no codable reply

7. WHAT YEAR IS IT (NOW)?
    Year _____
    Does not know
    No answer, no codable reply

Table 11.12 (cont)

Excerpt 2

1. HOW IS YOUR INTEREST IN THINGS? (DO YOU KEEP UP YOUR INTERESTS?)
   Interested
   Has less interest in things than is usual for him
   Severe, frequent or persistent loss in interest
   No answer, no codable reply

2. ARE YOU STILL INTERESTED IN YOUR CLOTHES AND HOW YOU LOOK?
   No loss of interest
   He neglects appearance
   Severe, frequent or persistent neglect
   No answer, no codable reply

3. WHAT HAVE YOU ENJOYED DOING RECENTLY? (HAS THERE BEEN ANY CHANGE?) (DID YOU USE TO ENJOY DOING THINGS?)
   Something named
   Almost nothing enjoyed
   Severe, frequent or persistent lack of enjoyment
   No answer, no codable reply

4. WHAT HAVE YOU BEEN DOING WITH YOUR FREE TIME? (If no active activities:) HAVE YOU LOST INTEREST RECENTLY?
   Mentions continued active activities
   He spends little of his free time at any form of active
      (such as bowling) recreational activity
   Has recently lost interest in active activities
   No answer, no codable reply

5. DO YOU WATCH TELEVISION OR LISTEN TO THE RADIO? (If no:) HAVE YOU LOST INTEREST RECENTLY?
   Mentions continued interest
   Spends little of his free time in any form of passive
      activities
   Has recently lost interest in television or radio
   No answer, no codable reply

6. Interviewer rating from Q1–5: Overall severity rating of loss of interest.
   Negligible
   Mild
   Moderate
   Severe
   Extreme
   No answers, no codable replies

Source: Henderson, Duncan-Jones and Finlay-Jones (1983)

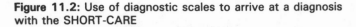

Figure 11.2: Use of diagnostic scales to arrive at a diagnosis with the SHORT-CARE

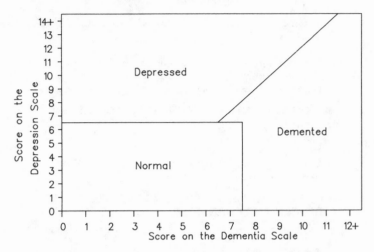

to arrive at a diagnosis as shown in Figure 11.2. Thus, elderly people with low scores on the depression and dementia scales are regarded as normal, while people with high scores are diagnosed as depressed or demented depending on which symptoms predominate. This approach has been found to agree well with psychiatrists' diagnoses of dementia and depression, yet has the virtue of great simplicity.

Cambridge Mental Disorders of the Elderly Examination (CAMDEX)

The CAMDEX (Roth *et al.*, in press) is the most recently developed of the standardised psychiatric examinations for the elderly. It has three main components: a psychiatric interview with the elderly person, a series of cognitive tests, and an interview with a relative or friend of the elderly person. In this respect, it is unlike the GMS and SHORT-CARE which basically comprise only the first of these components.

The psychiatric interview covers the elderly person's current physical and mental state, enquires about the history of any symptoms, and elicits information about problems in other family members. The cognitive testing incorporates the Mini-Mental State but adds many additional tests to cover cognitive deficits either not assessed in the Mini-Mental or only briefly covered. The third component, the interview with a relative or friend, asks about personality change and any cognitive deficits noted in everyday life. The first two components of the CAMDEX takes 40–60 minutes to complete, while the informant interview requires an additional 10 minutes.

The interviewer uses the information gathered in the CAMDEX to make a psychiatric diagnosis. However, the CAMDEX does not provide a computerised set of diagnostic rules of the sort provided for the GMS. Rather, the interviewer is left to apply traditional diagnostic criteria using the information gathered. Nevertheless, the CAMDEX does attempt to provide much more specific diagnoses than the earlier standardised examinations. Whereas they aimed only to diagnose dementia, the CAMDEX separates dementia into four categories: senile dementia of the Alzheimer type, multi-infarct dementia, mixed dementia, and dementia secondary to other cause. The CAMDEX also gathers information for the diagnosis of depression, delirium and other psychiatric disorders.

When two psychiatrists use the CAMDEX with the same patients they show good agreement in their diagnoses. The CAMDEX helps in this regard by ensuring that identical information is collected by different psychiatrists. However, the actual diagnostic decision rests very much on the psychiatrist's extensive clinical skills, rather than on the application of an unambiguous set of diagnostic rules, so this examination could not be used by anyone but a skilled clinician.

Although only in its youth, the CAMDEX represents a very promising approach. The direction it has taken, of incorporating information from sources other than a psychiatric interview with the elderly person, is also being adopted in a version of the GMS currently under development.

Management of Senile Dementia

INTRODUCTION

The common view that 'prevention is better than cure' applies as much to senile dementia as to any other disorder. However, even if dementia can eventually be prevented to a certain degree through modification of risk factors, there will still be very many cases developing. What can be done for these cases? Although it is unlikely that the disorders which produce dementia will be curable in the sense that demented people will recover lost abilities and return to their former selves, it is quite possible that in the near future there will be treatments to provide relief of symptoms and perhaps to slow down the course of the dementia. However, even without effective treatments, there is still much that can be done to make the lives of the demented person and his or her family as dignified and pleasant as possible.

The management of dementia necessarily varies as a function of the stage of the dementia. For example, elderly people with mild dementia will generally be able to live effectively in the community provided the demands of their daily life are not too great. With severe dementia, on the other hand, institutional care is a likely option, and will be a necessity where the elderly person is living alone. This chapter looks at the opportunities for management at various stages of dementia and ends with an overview of current treatment approaches.

RECOGNITION OF DEMENTIA

The first step in managing dementia must be to recognise its presence. Family members and friends may recognise that there is some cognitive impairment long before there is formal recognition of dementia by a medical practitioner. Medical recognition of the problem will generally be by the general practitioner or by staff in a hospital where the elderly person has been admitted for some other condition. With mild dementia, diagnosis is very difficult, even by specialists. However, even moderate cases are often missed by medical practitioners. In a famous Scottish study of the unreported needs of elderly people, Williamson and his colleagues (1964) found that as many as four out of five cases of dementia they diagnosed during home interviews were unrecognised by the person's family physician. Other community surveys of the elderly carried out in Wales (Parsons, 1965) and Germany (Weyerer, 1983) have found general practitioners to be somewhat better at recognising dementia in their patients, but they still missed around half the cases. On the other hand, these studies found that general practitioners hardly ever mistakenly diagnose a normal elderly person as demented. Because of the important role of the family physician in managing cases of dementia in the community, failure to recognise cases is unfortunate. However, there are simple means of improving recognition. For example, the Mini-Mental State Examination (see Chapter 11) takes only ten minutes to administer, and can be given by a trained nurse, yet it correctly detects close to 90 per cent of dementia and delirium cases (Anthony *et al.*, 1982).

Even without the availability of effective treatments, there are good reasons for attempting to recognise cases of dementia in the community. Firstly, family members will undoubtedly have seen the emergence of some disturbing behaviour, the reasons for which they have not understood. In such cases, it is natural to believe the elderly person's difficult behaviour is wilful. With an explanation of the brain changes which cause the behaviour, it becomes easier to understand and tolerate. Relatives also need to be prepared for what the future may hold, since their own lives may be drastically affected. A second reason for early recognition of dementia is that it can be made worse with certain types of medication. Alzheimer's disease, the major cause of dementia, involves a deficiency of the cholinergic system (see Chapter 4). Certain drugs have a disruptive effect on the cholinergic system, which may be of little consequence to a normal person but can greatly worsen a dementia. Recognition of dementia will also help the physician to understand and manage episodes of delirium, which are not uncommon in the demented. In these episodes, the person's confusion becomes greater, awareness of the environment is lessened, thought and language become incoherent, and the sleep–waking cycle may be disrupted.

Once dementia is recognised, in some cases it is worth seeking out possible treatable causes. A small minority of dementias are potentially treatable, for example, those due to abnormalities in the flow of cerebrospinal fluid in the brain, brain tumours, or disorders of the thyroid gland. In one study, 200 cases of dementia were thoroughly investigated and a potentially reversible cause was found in thirteen patients (Smith and Kiloh, 1981). Such potentially reversible dementias were, however, more likely in patients aged 45–64 (11 per cent of cases) than in the group aged 65 or over (only 4 per cent). The investigation procedures involved in finding potentially treatable dementias are very costly and it has been questioned whether it would be practical to thoroughly investigate all cases of senile dementia given the great numbers of patients involved and the small number of potentially treatable dementias likely to be found (Eastwood and Corbin, 1981). With the rarer middle-aged cases of dementia, however, thorough investigation is more likely to prove worthwhile.

COMMUNITY CARE FOR THE DEMENTED

Most demented people, particularly those with mild dementia, can continue to live in the general community with some assistance from relatives and from health and welfare services.

The demented living alone

For those who live alone, the problems are somewhat different than for those who live with families. As the elderly person's capabilities progressively decline, increasingly greater efforts are required to keep them living independently. Help can be provided to overcome physical limitations by modifying the living environment. For example, hand rails can be added to the bathroom and stairs to avoid falls. If gas appliances can cause difficulty by being accidentally left on, they can be converted to electricity. Even simple signs reminding the demented person to switch off appliances or to carry out certain cleaning tasks can be surprisingly effective. Electronic monitoring is useful to detect any emergency situation. In one such system, the elderly person wears a small device around the neck with a button which can be pushed if, for example, there is a serious fall. The device sends a radio signal to the person's telephone, a series of emergency numbers is dialled automatically and a prerecorded message played. In the future we can expect the development of computer-based systems which can detect any pattern of unusual activity in the home, such as lack of movement or appliances left on, with appropriate action being taken automatically.

Domiciliary services are of great value in maintaining demented elderly people in the community. These services include: community nurses, meals-on-wheels, home help, good neighbour schemes, day centres and day hospitals, and visits by a general practitioner. However, as a person's dementia worsens the point will be reached where the effort to maintain them in the community cannot be justified and institutional care must be considered. In fact, Bergmann and his colleagues (1978) found that in Britain much of the effort towards supporting demented people in the community went on those living alone, yet they often proved not to be viable for community living. They felt that services would be better redirected to those people supported by their families.

One difficult ethical problem that can arise is where the demented person living alone wishes to continue living independently, while relatives and neighbours who are alarmed at their behaviour believe that institutional care would be preferable. The issue comes down to whether demented people should be allowed to choose to live in a situation where they are at risk of injury. With elderly people who are physically frail but intellectually sound, it is easier to accept a choice of this sort, but demented people might be thought incapable of making an informed decision. According to this view, the demented person has a similar status to a child. We do not allow children to take risks freely because their understanding of such situations is poorer than that of adults. However, against this paternalistic view it can be argued that a demented elderly person who happily lives alone and as a result shortens his or her life by a few years is better off than one who lives a slightly longer but unhappier life in institutional care.

The demented living with relatives

For the demented person cared for by relatives, the welfare of the family is an important consideration. In Chapter 3, this issue was discussed at some length. Although institutional care is probably the best help for despairing relatives, there are many other supports available in the community.

In many countries there are now organisations which provide information and support to relatives of dementia sufferers as well as promoting research into the problem. These organisations go by different names in different countries: in Britain there is the Alzheimer's Disease Society, in the United States the Alzheimer's Disease and Related Disorders Association (ADRDA), and in Australia the Alzheimer's Disease and Related Disorders Society (ADARDS). In fact, there is now an Alzheimer's Disease International — the International Federation of Alzheimer's Disease and Related Disorders Societies. Another valuable source of advice for relatives is the book *The 36-hour Day* which is essentially a manual for care-givers. The information needed on services available for the demented differs from country to country, but this book is now available in a British edition (Mace *et al.*, 1985) as well as the original American edition (Mace and Rabins, 1981).

In recent years, support groups for relatives of the demented have become popular. In these groups, relatives caring for a demented person meet regularly to receive information and share experiences. At first, groups tend to focus on the needs of the demented person, but later emphasis shifts to the needs of the caregiver. To be able to attend such a group, a caregiver may require someone to look after the demented person for a period. Support groups should therefore be established in conjunction with a day-care or granny-sitting service. A recent study has shown that support groups can be effective (Kahan *et al.*, 1985). In this study, relatives attending a support group were compared to others who were on a waiting list to attend the group. After eight weekly group meetings, attenders were found to have a greater knowledge about dementia, to feel less burdened, and slightly less depressed than those on the waiting list.

Day hospitals and day-care services are an important facility for demented people living in the community. Day hospitals are basically medical in orientation and are attached to a hospital or health centre. The elderly person visits one or more times a week for assessment, treatment, or rehabilitation. However, the major function of day hospitals is not always as it is supposed to be. In an evaluation of a Scottish geriatric psychiatry day hospital, its main function was found to be short-term relief for family members until a long-stay bed became available for their demented relative (Greene and Timbury, 1979). Although day hospitals might be expected to reduce demand for inpatient care, studies of the effects of opening

120

them in Scotland found little change in the number of patients admitted to hospital or put on the waiting list for inpatient care (Greene and Timbury, 1979; Ballinger, 1984). Day-care facilities, by contrast, are non-medical and fulfil a more social function, providing recreational facilities and social support for elderly people and respite for their caregiving relatives.

Even when family members are keen to care for a demented relative, the point may come where the cost to them is too great and institutional care must be considered. The decision to seek institutional care can be a difficult one, with caregivers feeling a desire for relief after years of strain yet regarding the necessity to institutionalise their loved one as a sign of failure. The family physician can do much to help matters by broaching the subject of institutional care when the strain appears too great. An ethical problem arises when the caregiving relatives seek institutional care, while the elderly person is opposed to any move. The situation here is rather different from where the demented person lives alone, because their decision will affect the relatives as well as themselves. In this case, following the demented person's wishes is harder to justify because of the great cost to others.

INSTITUTIONAL CARE FOR THE DEMENTED

Institutional care facilities for the elderly go by somewhat different names in different countries, but are generally distinguished by the level of nursing care they provide. However, labels like *nursing home* or *hospital* are often not helpful in describing a type of institutional care because such a diversity of facilities and approaches can be found under the one rubric. This section examines some of the important factors determining quality of care across all types of institutions.

Type of environment

Institutionalisation can have a bad effect on the demented. In one Swiss study (Brull, Wertheimer and Haller, 1979), demented people were followed over several years to track the course of their cognitive decline. Some of these people remained stable over many years, whereas others declined dramatically. Those demented people who were admitted to a nursing home were found to be more likely to decline than those who remained at home or were admitted to a hospital. The authors commented:

> It seems reasonable to suppose that the placing of a patient in a nursing home encouraged a kind of withdrawal and contributed to the deterioration of the most vulnerable subgroup . . . It acts in this way through its implicit connotation that the patients are being set aside by society and because of the diminution of every kind of stimulus, in contrast to their previous lives, whether they were at home or whether they were in a hospital milieu operated on the basis of a policy of rehabilitation (p. 204).

Although there is no research on what type of environment is best for the demented, it is possible to make some recommendations on the basis of a general knowledge of the cognitive limitations present in dementia. Demented people have problems adjusting to a changing environment because of their difficulties in learning. Once they move into an institution, basic knowledge acquired over many years in their own home may no longer be relevant (for example how to find the toilet) and new knowledge must be acquired. An example of this is a lady admitted to a home where she began urinating on the floor every night instead of using the commode chair (even though a light was on). The woman's daughter was asked to re-arrange the furniture in the room exactly as it had been in the woman's own home, with the result that she immediately started using the commode (Marshall and Eaton, 1980). Of course, admission to an institution must inevitably require some new learning. A stable, predictable environment is more likely to aid learning and avoid unnecessary agitation. When first admitted to an institution, demented people are slow to regard it as home. They can be continually agitated because they wish to leave for their former home, but are unable to do so. Only with time and predictability is a new routine and feeling of belonging established.

A stable, predictable environment is not the same as one where no choices are available. Providing choices may be very important in preventing apathetic and passive behaviour in demented people. However, for the demented, choices available must be appropriate to their cognitive limitations. They are capable of choosing, for example, whether they wish to have afternoon tea or attend a recreational activity, but other choices may not be appropriate because they are based on false beliefs or faulty reasoning. The general importance of providing choices to elderly people in institutions is dramatically illustrated by an experiment carried out in an American nursing home (Langer and Rodin, 1976). One floor of this home was selected for a brief programme to increase personal responsibility, while another floor was used for comparison. The 'personal responsibility' floor was given a talk by the nursing home administrator where he emphasised the choices residents had available to them. Residents were told they could rearrange their furniture, visit friends on other floors, choose various recreational activities, and were encouraged to make complaints about any aspect of the home they wanted changed. Each resident was also given a gift of a small plant to look after. The residents on the 'comparison' floor were also given a similar talk, but this time it emphasised the staff's responsibility for the residents, rather than the residents' responsibility for themselves. The residents were also given plants, but they were looked after for them by the staff. Over the following weeks, residents on both floors were studied. The residents on the 'personal responsibility' floor assessed themselves as happier and as having greater control over their lives compared to those on the 'comparison' floor. Staff believed these residents to be more alert, and they were observed spending more time interacting with other residents and staff. A follow-up 18 months later showed lasting effects. In fact, the mortality rate of residents on the 'personal responsibility' floor was only half that of residents on the 'comparison' floor (Rodin and Langer, 1977). This experiment shows that even small efforts to increase choice and control can bring noticeable improvements in residents' quality of life. It must be noted that the residents in this experiment were all mobile and communicative, so none would have been severely demented. However, there is every reason to expect that choice and control are as important to elderly people with mild-to-moderate mental impairments as to those with physical impairments.

Segregation of the demented

Institutional care is needed by the elderly with physical disabilities as well as those with cognitive deficits. A heated issue is whether both groups should be mixed together or segregated into separate types of institutions. Arguments can be made for both approaches. Integrationists point out that it is undesirable for the demented to mix only with other demented people because this could make their confusion worse. Furthermore, once a person is placed in a special-purpose institution for the demented, there is a labelling and stigma which may adversely influence how that person is treated. For example, they may be regarded as beyond hope and little will be done to stimulate them. Segregation, on the other hand, can be regarded as desirable because institutions can have special design features and programmes to suit the demented. A major argument in favour of segregation is that it is unfair to the physically frail to mix them with the demented. The disturbed behaviour of demented residents can badly affect the morale of the rational residents.

Despite the importance of the issue of segregation versus integration, little research has been done on it. The one exception is a book by Meacher (1972) in which he studied three British nursing homes described as 'separatist' and three described as 'ordinary'. Despite the contrasting labels given to these homes, only 58 per cent of the residents in the separatist homes were mentally confused, compared to 16 per cent in the ordinary homes. Meacher found a reduced quality of life in the separatist homes. For example, complaints about confused behaviour were more common in the separatist homes, particularly from the rational residents. Although Meacher's book is often seen as providing strong evidence against segregation, it can perhaps be better viewed as showing the undesirability of mixing demented and non-demented residents in roughly equal proportions. Meacher's ordinary homes appear to provide a better example of the effects of segregation than his so-called separatist ones.

The problems which integration can cause for rational residents are poignantly recorded in a diary published by a physically frail, but intellectually sound, elderly woman of her experiences in several Australian nursing homes (Newton, 1979). At one point in her diary, she sums up her feelings in the following memorable words:

Men and women with terminal illness may have hardened arteries and creaking joints, but their minds are in no way crippled. For them to be enclosed in nursing homes where night and day senility, with its apathy, strident garrulity, and frequently painful psychiatric problems must call the tune for everyone, can only be a living death (p. 106).

The issue of segregation is perhaps best not seen in terms of demented versus rational, but of disturbed versus normal behaviour. Severely demented people in institutions will typically be immobile, incontinent and uncommunicative. At this stage of their dementia, they are basically a physical nursing problem. They are not difficult to manage and do not disturb other residents. However, in earlier stages of dementia, there may be aimless, confused wandering which will be disturbing to other residents. The confused wanderer may move from room to room interfering with other people's possessions and annoying them with repetitive and senseless talk. Segregation appears to be a desirable option at this stage of dementia, with integration becoming possible once again when the dementia progresses and physical nursing care is the basic requirement. Such behaviour can be more readily tolerated in an environment specially designed to cope with it.

Even more disturbed behaviour can arise as a phase of dementia in a minority of cases. These may require specialist psychiatric care. Published data on referrals to one British psychiatric service from old people's homes revealed the following as the major problem behaviours (in order of frequency):

(1) Agitated, restless, interfering behaviour
(2) Aggression
(3) Socially unacceptable behaviour (such as masturbating in public or urinating on other residents)
(4) Subjective suffering
(5) Repeated questions and need for reassurance
(6) Uncooperativeness
(7) Wandering
(8) Complaining and refusing to conform
(9) Noisiness

Dementia was the cause of these problem behaviours in most cases, but other psychiatric problems sometimes caused difficulties (Margo, Robinson and Corea, 1980).

Architectural features

One of the benefits of segregation is that facilities can be specifically designed to take account of the limitations of demented residents. The architectural requirements of the demented are somewhat different from those of the physically frail, yet often facilities are designed primarily with physical impairments in mind.

Some very useful design principles have been presented by Henderson (1980). He attempts to overcome the problems caused by

125

wandering by providing corridors as circular return routes rather than with dead ends. Similarly, pathways in an external garden can be of a circular design with seats and points of interest (such as ponds, bird baths) along the way. Rather than use fences to prevent wandering outside the grounds, he advocates a physical barrier such as low shrubs planted in a sloping ditch, which does not restrict vision of the street. This creates an effect of open freedom, while still containing the wanderer. Exit gates from the grounds can be planned so as not to be visible to residents, lest they stimulate the desire to escape.

Choosing the correct door to a bedroom can be a problem for the demented. This can be aided by use of a special bright colour for each resident, the person's name on the door in large letters, and perhaps a photograph. Similarly, toilet doors can be painted a bright distinctive colour with a recognisable symbol. Doors which are for staff use only can be camouflaged to discourage resident use.

Room fittings can be designed to retain features familiar to elderly people. For example, older-style taps in the bathroom and furniture in the bedroom will cause less confusion than modern fittings. Free-standing furniture in the bedroom is desirable because it allows rearrangement to suit the habits of each resident.

Confused night wandering can be a problem with the demented. This problem seems to be due to a lack of visual input at night. It has been found that this same type of behaviour can be induced in the daytime by placing the demented person in a darkened room (Cameron, 1941). Presumably, demented people find it difficult to remember the spatial features of their environment without some visual input. To overcome this problem, night lighting of bedrooms and corridors is important. By providing dim lighting in corridors and brighter lighting in destinations, such as toilets, it is possible to guide residents to appropriate places.

Normalisation

Although segregation may be undesirable to the extent that it isolates the demented from the normal world of the rational, much of this disadvantage can be overcome by attempts to normalise the institutional environment. *Normalisation* refers to attempts to make the living environment of handicapped people as close as possible to that of the general community. Normalisation programmes for the demented can take the form of placing them in ordinary houses, in family-sized groupings, under the direction of a supervisor (Marshall and Eaton, 1980). From the outside, such facilities look no different from ordinary family dwellings. Inside, bedrooms can be individualised, with the resident's own personal furniture arranged as they wish. Residents can help with simple kitchen chores and household maintenance. Interaction with the rest of the community can be maintained in many ways, for example, by attending day centres or through regular outings.

Normalisation programmes of this sort are most appropriate for mild-to-moderately demented people who require minimal physical nursing care. In severe dementia, physical nursing requirements and an inability to communicate at the most basic level must necessarily divorce the life of the demented person from that of the general community. Normalisation is also difficult for demented people with severe behavioural disturbances which will disrupt any attempts at community living.

Staff morale

Working with the demented in institutions is a demanding occupation. Although in recent years there has been much attention given to the strain on family members of caring for a demented person in the community, similar strains must arise for staff involved in institutional care. Many people involved in care of the demented advocate part-time work in the area as being more desirable than full-time work. They believe that staff can seldom cope with such demanding work on a full-time basis. Fortunately, attempts to improve the quality of life for demented residents of institutions may also have positive benefits for staff morale.

DRUG TREATMENTS

Numerous drugs have been tried as treatments for senile dementia, but few have been extensively evaluated. Two approaches will be looked at here. One is an older treatment which is still in use, and the other is a recent approach based on discoveries about brain function in Alzheimer's disease. Neither approach aims to cure dementia, but to relieve some of its ill-effects.

127

Metabolic enhancers

It will be recalled that senile dementia was once thought to be due to a narrowing of blood vessels with the consequence that there was an inadequate supply of blood to the brain. To overcome this blood supply problem, drugs which increase blood flow were tried as treatments. These drugs, called *vasodilators*, were expected to work by widening the blood vessels. Although the theory of inadequate blood supply is now discredited, vasodilators are still sometimes used in the treatment of senile dementia. The most widely used vasodilator is dihydroergotoxine which is marketed under the brand name of Hydergine. In recent years, researchers have come to recognise that drugs like Hydergine do not only increase blood flow, they also enhance the process by which the brain derives energy (Reisberg, 1981). Accordingly, such drugs have been renamed as *metabolic enhancers*.

Many studies have evaluated the effectiveness of Hydergine in the treatment of senile dementia. The usual approach is to have one group of patients receive Hydergine while another group receives a placebo. It is also important that the people administering the pills do not know which patients are receiving the drug and which the placebo, otherwise, they may convey greater expectation of improvement to the patients receiving the drug and might also be biased in their observations of the drug's effects. In studies which meet these rigorous requirements, Hydergine is generally found to have some effect, although the improvement is not spectacular. Furthermore, the improvement seems to be greater in the area of mood than of cognitive function (Cole and Liptzin, 1984). Researchers have not specifically looked at whether Hydergine differs in its effectiveness for Alzheimer's disease or multi-infarct dementia. However, one authority believes that studies which tested the drug predominantly on cases of Alzheimer's disease found greater improvements (Reisberg, 1981).

Cholinergic enhancement

During the 1970s, the important discovery that Alzheimer's disease involves a deficit of the cholinergic system was made. This discovery led to the hope that a drug treatment might be developed to enhance the functioning of the cholinergic system. The most popular approach tried was based on an analogy with the successful

128

treatment of Parkinson's disease. Parkinson's disease is known to involve a deficiency of the neurons which use dopamine as a neurotransmitter. By administering a drug which the body uses to make dopamine, it was found that the symptoms of Parkinson's disease could be relieved. With Alzheimer's disease, many attempts have been made to increase the supply of the neurotransmitter acetylcholine by administering drugs which the body uses to manufacture it. Two such drugs have been tried. The first is *choline*, which is the actual chemical used by the body, and the other is *lecithin*, which is a dietary source of choline. Choline proved less popular because some patients given it developed an unpleasant fishy smell which led them to be socially ostracised! The more popular alternative, lecithin, is of course readily available in health food shops. Its only side-effect appears to be occasional stomach upsets and diarrhoea. Over the many evaluation studies which have been carried out, the effects of choline and lecithin have proved disappointing. In general, these treatments have had no effect on cognitive deficits, although there may be some small improvements in late-onset Alzheimer's disease patients when the dosages are carefully tailored to suit the individual (Little *et al.*, 1985; Jorm, 1986c).

A second approach to enhancing the cholinergic system involves drugs which inhibit the enzyme which breaks down acetylcholine. In contrast to choline and lecithin treatments, which aim to increase the manufacture of acetylcholine, these treatments aim to reduce its destruction. Two drugs which have this effect have been tried, *physostigmine* and *THA*. THA has the advantage of having a longer-acting effect than physostigmine, but it has been much less widely studied. Until recent years, physostigmine could only be administered by injection, which severely limited its usefulness. However, there has now been developed a version of this drug which can be taken by mouth. Physostigmine is a drug with a narrow 'therapeutic window', which means it is effective at only a small range of doses. If the dose is too low physostigmine has little effect, while if it is too high the drug can actually worsen cognitive function. Furthermore, the 'too low' dose is very close to the 'too high' dose, and the optimal dosage varies widely from individual to individual. For this reason, it is not sensible to give one group of Alzheimer patients a certain dose of physostigmine and another group a placebo. For some patients, the particular dosage chosen may be too low, for others too high, and for some lucky ones it may be optimal. In fact, studies which have evaluated physostigmine and THA using the same dosage for every patient find no overall benefit. However,

129

when an effort is made to first determine the optimal dosage of the drug for each patient, physostigmine and THA appear to produce some small improvement in cognitive function (Jorm, 1986c).

A third approach to enhancing the cholinergic system in Alzheimer's disease is to combine physostigmine with either choline or lecithin. This combination approach tries to increase acetylcholine levels by simultaneously boosting its production and blocking its destruction. Only a few studies have evaluated this approach, but those that have individually tailored the dosage of physostigmine used in combination with choline or lecithin have produced encouraging results (Jorm, 1986c). The combination approach appears to be the most promising of the cholinergic enhancement treatments so far; however, it has been tried on only a small number of patients and is still very much an experimental treatment.

Cholinergic enhancement treatments are still in their early stages. Improved drugs which affect this neurotransmitter system will be developed in coming years and offer promise of useful effects. However, dramatic improvements should not be expected. Alzheimer's disease involves actual loss of cholinergic neurons, so there is a limit to what can be achieved by boosting the chemical processes which take place in these neurons. Furthermore, other neurotransmitters are known to be involved in Alzheimer's disease, particularly in early-onset cases, so it may be necessary for a cocktail of drugs to be carefuly tailored to the individual patient to get the best results.

PSYCHOLOGICAL INTERVENTIONS

There are two broad kinds of psychological interventions which can be carried out with the demented elderly. The first approach views the demented person as having certain psychological deficits which must be changed if they are to function in their environment. In this approach, the aim is to change the person so they better fit this environment. The second approach regards the demented person's environment as making inappropriate demands on his or her limited cognitive capacities. The environment is therefore changed to better fit these remaining capacities. To give an example of these contrasting approaches, imagine an elderly demented man who lives in a nursing home and who has trouble finding his way to the toilet. One approach to this problem would be to change the person by giving him some special training in finding the toilet. An alternative would be to change the environment by painting a distinctive red line from the man's room to the toilet and also painting the toilet door the same colour. In practice, of course, both approaches are often closely intertwined in psychological interventions.

Within both these broad approaches, psychological interventions can aim to overcome different areas of deficit. An important aim is to improve cognitive functions such as memory. A second area of deficit is that of social interaction and apathy. As the specific sorts of interventions appropriate for overcoming cognitive and social deficits differ we will examine these two areas of deficit separately.

Overcoming cognitive deficits

Treatments which aim to improve cognitive function by directly changing the demented person have not been popular. However, there have been a few attempts of this sort. One approach involves training demented people to encode information in memory more effectively. In Chapter 5 it was shown that encoding of information into long-term memory is deficient in Alzheimer's disease patients. In normal people, encoding of word lists can be improved greatly by the use of imagery. As an example, say that the following list of words had to be remembered: cat, apple, sky, scissors, lawn. These could be linked together using visual images in various ways. For example, visualise a *cat* eating an *apple*; suddenly, the apple flies from the cat's mouth up to the blue *sky* where a giant pair of *scissors* cuts it in half; the two halves fall down to the ground and land on a *lawn*. Although these images seem ridiculous, once the words are so linked they become very easy to retrieve, as the reader can readily demonstrate by attempting to recall the list using the first word, *cat*, as a cue. Another method of improving encoding is to concentrate primarily on the meanings (rather than the sounds or spellings) of the words which have to be remembered. This could be done, for example, by making a definition of each word or by associating each with words of similar meaning. One study has evaluated the effectiveness of training in such encoding strategies with demented elderly people (Brinkman *et al.*, 1982). The training was found to produce a slight improvement in memory for lists of words. However, it is doubtful that this type of training is useful in everyday memory situations where lists of words rarely have to be remembered. Even where lists are involved, as in shopping, people prefer to write things down rather than use techniques like imagery.

Memory aids

Another approach involving changing the demented person is to train them to use memory aids such as a diary. The aim here is to improve retrieval from long-term memory by providing better retrieval strategies. One attempt of this sort (Hanley and Lusty, 1984) involved providing an elderly demented woman with a watch and a diary containing personal information and daily appointments. Very little improvement was noted until specific training was given in how to use the watch and diary. Then, using the diary, the woman was able to answer many questions about herself which were previously beyond her and she began to keep some appointments. Improvement was somewhat hampered by the fact that she frequently lost the diary! However, once training was discontinued, the woman rapidly lost the skills she had gained.

Reality orientation

A major limitation of attempts to change demented people is that these require a high degree of active involvement and new learning by the demented person. We saw in Chapter 5 that early in dementia the capacity for the kind of effortful cognitive processes involved in novel situations is lost, while more practised and automated processes are better retained. Unfortunately, psychological interventions which attempt to change the person rely heavily on effortful processing. For this reason, interventions which change the environment to fit the demented person's capabilities may be more profitable.

Undoubtedly the most popular of the approaches which rely primarily on environmental change is *reality orientation*. This approach was developed for use with the demented elderly in the United States during the 1960s and its use has since spread widely. The aim of reality orientation is to assist the demented elderly living in institutions to overcome their confusion and disorientation. It is not unusual for demented people living in institutions such as nursing homes not to know where they are, what time of day or night it is, the season, or the year. Reality orientation programmes involve using every contact by staff as an opportunity for overcoming this sort of disorientation. For example, if a nurse was going to help an old lady dress she would not say: 'Time to get dressed now, dear', but something like:

Good morning, Mrs Smith. I'm Sister Brown the nurse. It's 8 o'clock in the morning now. That's the time you get changed out of your nightie and into your dress. After you're dressed you'll be able to go off to the craft room and Mrs Johnson will take care of you there.

As well as these 24 hours-a-day attempts to overcome disorientation, there are special reality orientation classes held each day. These last around 30 minutes, involve only a handful of patients at a time, and take place in a classroom setting. In a class, an instructor reinforces basic orientation knowledge by going over his or her name, the patients' names, the location, the day, month and year etc. Patients may be asked to read such information aloud from a board and then to write it down for themselves. With less confused patients, the emphasis might be on topics such as forthcoming visits of relatives, approaching holidays, discussion of current events, and plans for social get-togethers. As well, the ward or home will have large clocks, calendars, and schedules of daily events placed in strategic places to further orient the patients. Basically, reality orientation attempts a reorganisation of the demented person's living environment so as to provide greater opportunities for encoding and retrieval of orientation information.

Many studies have compared the effects of reality orientation to standard institutional practice. In most studies, only the effectiveness of reality orientation classes (without 24-hour reality orientation) has been evaluated. It appears to be very difficult to implement a 24 hour-a-day reality orientation programme successfully, perhaps because of the demands it puts on busy nursing staff. Reality orientation classes alone do seem to have a small effect on dementia patients' orientation, but the effect is not large enough to be useful. However, when 24-hour reality orientation is implemented, the effects are much better (Harris and Ivory, 1976; Citrin and Dixon, 1977). Despite this success, there has been some questioning of the appropriateness of the goals of reality orientation. It has been suggested that it is not really all that important for demented elderly people living in institutions to know what day and month it is (Powell-Proctor and Miller, 1982). Rather, they need basic self-care skills like dressing, bathing, and going to the toilet unaided. Unfortunately, such skills are ignored in reality orientation programmes.

Overcoming social deficits

Apathy and lack of social interaction are characteristic of moderate and severe dementia. Some psychological interventions aim to overcome these deficiencies. At least in part, apathy amongst demented people living in institutions may be a reaction to a lack of opportunity for activity. It has been shown that activity levels can be increased greatly by providing suitable recreational materials (Jenkins *et al.*, 1977), and even more so by providing encouragement in their use (Burton, 1980).

Token economy

An important type of intervention aimed at social deficits is the *token economy*. Token economies were first used to motivate chronic psychotic patients in psychiatric hospitals but have since been extended to many other groups, including the demented elderly. In a token economy, plastic tokens are given out by staff when patients engage in constructive activities. These tokens can then be spent on various extra privileges. In one token economy for the demented (Mishara, 1978), tokens were given for social interaction with other patients, doing work on the ward, carrying out self-care activities, and good personal hygiene. Tokens could be exchanged for such things as cigarettes, wine, permission to leave the ward, and extra food. After 6 months under a token economy, some demented patients were found to engage in fewer bizarre and unusual behaviours and to have decreased incontinence. Others, however, showed no change. Interestingly, though, similar changes were found in a ward which did not use the token economy, but simply attempted to improve the demented patients' living conditions. This was done by providing more activities and social stimulation, increasing the patients' opportunities to make choices in daily activities, and promoting an awareness amongst staff that they should be working for the patients' benefit rather than simply running an efficient ward. Highly structured programmes like the token economy may not be necessary to reduce socially inappropriate behaviour in the demented elderly.

To some people, programmes like the token economy are repugnant. It seems to involve coercing people to engage in activities that they might otherwise not choose. Indeed, it might well be asked whether demented people should be left alone to be apathetic and socially isolated if that is what they want. The moral issue involved here is a difficult one. The demented cannot clearly communicate to us whether they prefer to be apathetic or involved, so we must make a decision for them. Miller (1977) has stated the argument in favour of intervention so well that I can do no better than quote him:

> In work with handicapped individuals, of any type or age and in the absence of contrary evidence, it must be assumed that they will enjoy the best quality of life when they approach as near as is possible to the kind of life they would have lived if they had not suffered their handicaps. There is evidence that normal, elderly people still retain a need for some active involvement and participation in life . . . and none that they are happiest when totally abdicating their independence to an institution. The assumption must therefore be that the handicapped elderly, whatever the nature of their handicaps, will attain the highest possible quality of life when they get closest to functioning in an adequate and normal manner (p. 82)

Although the changes produced by psychological interventions are not major, it is encouraging to know that such changes are possible in dementia. It is easy to assume that the demented are incapable of improvement through such means. Through a better understanding of the cognitive strengths and weaknesses of the demented, it will undoubtedly be possible to produce better psychological interventions in the future.

References

Aho, K., Harmsen, P., Hatano, S., Marquardsen, J., Smirnov, V.E. and Strasser, T. (1980) Cerebrovascular disease in the community: results of a WHO collaborative study. *Bulletin of the World Health Organization*, *58*, 113–30

Åkesson, H.O. (1969) A population study of senile and arteriosclerotic psychoses. *Human Heredity*, *19*, 546–66

Albert, M., Naeser, M.A., Levine, H.L. and Garney, A.J. (1984) CT density numbers in patients with senile dementia of the Alzheimer's type. *Archives of Neurology*, *41*, 1264–9

Alexander, D.A. (1973) Some tests of intelligence and learning for elderly psychiatric patients: a validation study. *British Journal of Social and Clinical Psychology*, *12*, 188–93

Alter, M. (1967) Dermatoglyphic analysis as a diagnostic tool. *Medicine*, *46*, 35–56

Alzheimer, A. (1907) Über eine eigenartige Erkrankung der Hirnrinde. *Allgemeine Zeitschrift für Psychiatrie und Psychisch-Gerichtlich Medicin*, *64*, 146–8

Amaducci, L.S., Fratiglioni, L., Rocca, W.A., Fieschi, C., Livrea, P., Pedone, D. *et al.* (1985) Risk factors for Alzheimer's disease (AD): a case-control study on an Italian population. *Neurology*, *35*, 277

American Psychiatric Association (1980) *Diagnostic and statistical manual of mental disorders (3rd edition) DSM-III*, American Psychiatric Association, Washington, DC

Anthony, J.C., Le Resche, L., Niaz, U., Von Korff, M.R. and Folstein, M.F. (1982) Limits of the 'Mini-Mental State' as a screening test for dementia and delirium among hospital patients. *Psychological Medicine*, *12*, 397–408

Argyle, N., Jestice, S. and Brook, C.P.B. (1985) Psychogeriatric patients: their supporters' problems. *Age and Ageing*, *14*, 355–60

Baddeley, A.D. (1982) Domains of recollection. *Psychological Review*, *89*, 708–29

Ball, M.J., Fisman, M., Hachinski, V., Blume, W., Fox, A., Kral, V.A., Kirshen, A.J. and Fox, H. (1985) A new definition of Alzheimer's disease: a hippocampal dementia. *Lancet*, *1*, 14–16

Ballinger, B.R. (1984) The effects of opening a geriatric psychiatry day hospital. *Acta Psychiatrica Scandinavica*, *70*, 400–3

Barnes, R.F., Raskind, M.A., Scott, M. and Murphy, C. (1981) Problems of families caring for Alzheimer patients: use of a support group. *Journal of the American Geriatrics Society*, *29*, 80–5

Bayles, K.A. and Boone, D.R. (1982) The potential of language tasks for identifying senile dementia. *Journal of Speech and Hearing Disorders*, *47*, 210–17

Beal, M.F., Mazurek, M.F., Tran, V.T., Chattha, G., Bird, E.D. and Martin, J.B. (1985) Reduced numbers of somatostatin receptors in the cerebral cortex in Alzheimer's disease. *Science*, *229*, 289–91

Bedford, P.D. (1959) General medical aspects of confusional states in elderly people. *British Medical Journal, 2,* 185–8

Benson, D.F., Kuhl, D.E., Hawkins, R.A., Phelps, M.E., Cummings, J.L. and Tsai, S.Y. (1983) The fluorodeoxyglucose 18F scan in Alzheimer's disease and multi-infarct dementia. *Archives of Neurology, 40,* 711–14

Bergmann, K., Foster, E.M., Justice, A.W. and Matthews, V. (1978) Management of the demented elderly patient in the community. *British Journal of Psychiatry, 132,* 441–9

Besson, J.A.O., Corrigan, F.M., Foreman, E.I., Ashcroft, G.W., Eastwood, L.M. and Smith, F.W. (1983) Differentiating senile dementia of Alzheimer type and multi-infarct dementia by proton NMR imaging. *Lancet, 2,* 789

Blazer, D.G., Federspiel, C.F., Ray, W.A. and Schaffner, W. (1983) The risk of anticholinergic toxicity in the elderly: a study of prescribing practices in two populations. *Journal of Gerontology, 38,* 31–5

Bondareff, W. (1983) Age and Alzheimer disease. *Lancet, 1,* 1447

Bondareff, W., Baldy, R. and Levy, R. (1981) Quantitative computed tomography in senile dementia. *Archives of General Psychiatry, 38,* 1365–8

Brinkman, S.D., Smith, R.C., Meyer, J.S., Vroulis, G., Shaw, T., Gordon, J.R. and Allen, R.H. (1982) Lecithin and memory training in suspected Alzheimer's disease. *Journal of Gerontology, 37,* 4–9

Brull, J., Wertheimer, J. and Haller, E. (1979) Evolutive profiles in senile dementia. A psychological and neuropsychological longitudinal study. In F. Hoffmeister and C. Müller (eds) *Brain function in old age,* Springer-Verlag, Berlin

Burton, M. (1980) Evaluation and change in a psychogeriatric ward through direct observation and feedback. *British Journal of Psychiatry, 137,* 566–71

Buschke, H. and Fuld, P.A. (1974) Evaluating storage, retention, and retrieval in disordered memory and learning. *Neurology, 24,* 1019–25

Carr, A.C., Wilson, S.L., Ghosh, A., Ancill, R.J. and Woods, R.T. (1982) Automated testing of geriatric patients using a microcomputer-based system. *International Journal of Man-Machine Studies, 17,* 297–300

Caine, E.D. (1981) Pseudodementia. Current concepts and future directions. *Archives of General Psychiatry, 38,* 1359–64

Cameron, D.E. (1941) Studies in senile nocturnal delirium. *Psychiatric Quarterly, 15,* 47–53

Campbell, A.J., McCosh, L.M., Reinken, J. and Allan, B.C. (1983) Dementia in old age and the need for services. *Age and Ageing, 12,* 11–16

Christie, A.B. (1982) Changing patterns in mental illness in the elderly. *British Journal of Psychiatry, 140,* 154–9

Christie, A.B. and Train, J.D. (1984) Change in the pattern of care for the demented. *British Journal of Psychiatry, 144,* 9–15

Citrin, R.S. and Dixon, D.N. (1977) Reality orientation: a milieu therapy used in an institution for the aged. *Gerontologist, 17,* 39–43

Cole, J.O. and Liptzin, B. (1984) Drug treatment of dementia in the elderly. In D.W. Kay and G.D. Burrows (eds), *Handbook of studies on psychiatry and old age,* Elsevier, Amsterdam

137

REFERENCES

Copeland, J.R., Kelleher, M.J., Kellett, J.M., Gourlay, A.J., Gurland, B.J., Fleiss, J.L. and Sharpe, L. (1976) A semi-structured clinical interview for the assessment of diagnosis and mental state in the elderly: the Geriatric Mental State Schedule I. Development and reliability. *Psychological Medicine, 6,* 439–49

Corkin, S. (1982) Some relationships between global amnesias and the memory impairments in Alzheimer's disease. In S. Corkin *et al.* (eds) *Alzheimer's disease: a report of progress, (Aging,* Vol. 19), Raven Press, New York

Coyle, J.T., Price, D.L. and DeLong, M.R. (1983) Alzheimer's disease: a disorder of cortical cholinergic innervation. *Science, 219,* 1184–90

Cummings, J.L. and Benson, D.F. (1983) *Dementia: a clinical approach,* Butterworths, Boston

De Souza, E.B., Whitehouse, P.J., Kuhar, M.J., Price, D.L. and Vale, W.W. (1986) Reciprocal changes in corticotropin-releasing factor (CRF)-like immunoreactivity and CRF receptors in cerebral cortex of Alzheimer's disease. *Nature, 319,* 593–5

Diesfeldt, H.F.A., van Houte, L.R. and Moerkens, R.M. (1986) Duration of survival in senile dementia. *Acta Psychiatrica Scandinavica, 73,* 366–71

Doobov, A. (1980) *Relative costs of home care and nursing home and hospital care in Australia,* Australian Government Publishing Service, Canberra

Drachman, D.A. and Leavitt, J. (1974) Human memory and the cholinergic system: a relationship to aging? *Archives of Neurology, 30,* 113–21

Eastwood, R. and Corbin, S. (1981) Investigation of suspect dementia. *Lancet, 1,* 1261

Erkinjuntti, T., Sulkava, R. and Tilvis, R. (1985) HDL-cholesterol in dementia. *Lancet, 2,* 43

Evans, J.G. (1982) The psychiatric aspects of physical disease. In R. Levy and F. Post (eds), *The psychiatry of late life,* Blackwell Scientific Publications, Oxford

Folstein, M.F., Folstein, S.E. and McHugh, P.R. (1975) 'Mini-Mental State'. A practical method for grading the cognitive state of patients for the clinician. *Journal of Psychiatric Research, 12,* 189–98

Folstein, M.F. and McHugh, P.R. (1978) Dementia syndrome of depression. In R. Katzman, R.D. Terry and K.L. Bick (eds), *Alzheimer's disease: senile dementia and related disorders, (Aging,* Vol. 7), Raven Press, New York

Foster, N.L., Chase, T.N., Mansi, L., Brooks, R., Fedio, P., Patronas, N.J. and Di Chiro, G. (1984) Cortical abnormalities in Alzheimer's disease. *Annals of Neurology, 16,* 649–54

French, L.R., Schuman, L.M., Mortimer, J.A., Hutton, J.T., Boatman, R.A. and Christians, B. (1985) A case-control study of dementia of the Alzheimer type. *American Journal of Epidemiology, 121(3),* 414–21

Fuld, P.A. (1983) Psychometric differentiation of the dementias: an overview. In B. Reisberg (ed.), *Alzheimer's disease: the standard reference,* The Free Press, New York

Gajdusek, D.C. (1977) Unconventional viruses and the origin and disappearance of kuru. *Science, 197,* 943–60

Gajdusek, D.C. (1985) Hypothesis: interference with axonal transport of neurofilament as a common pathogenetic mechanism in certain diseases of the central nervous system. *New England Journal of Medicine, 312,* 714–19

Garraway, W.M., Whisnant, J.P., Furlan, A.J., Phillips, L.H., Kurland, L.T. and O'Fallon, M. (1979) The declining incidence of stroke. *New England Journal of Medicine, 300,* 449–52

Geddes, J.W., Monaghan, D.T., Cotman, C.W., Lott, I.T., Kim, R.C. and Chui, H.C. (1985) Plasticity of hippocampal circuitry in Alzheimer's disease. *Science, 230,* 1179–81

Gibson, A.J. and Kendrick, D.C. (1979) *The Kendrick Battery for the Detection of Dementia in the Elderly,* NFER-Nelson, Windsor, Berks

Gilhooly, M.L.M. (1984) The impact of care-giving on care-givers: factors associated with the psychological well-being of people supporting a dementing relative in the community. *British Journal of Medical Psychology, 57,* 35–44

Gilleard, C.J., Belford, H., Gilleard, E., Whittick, J.E. and Gledhill, K. (1984) Emotional distress amongst the supporters of the elderly mentally infirm. *British Journal of Psychiatry, 145,* 172–7

Golden, R.R., Teresi, J.A. and Gurland, B.A. (1983) Detection of dementia and depression cases with the Comprehensive Assessment and Referral Evaluation Interview Schedule. *International Journal of Aging and Human Development, 16,* 241–54

Greene, J.G., Smith, R., Gardiner, M. and Timbury, G.C. (1982) Measuring behavioural disturbance of elderly demented patients in the community and its effects on relatives: a factor analytic study. *Age and Ageing, 11,* 121–6

Greene, J.G. and Timbury, G.C. (1979) A geriatric psychiatry day hospital service: a five-year review. *Age and Ageing, 8,* 49–53

Gruenberg, E.M. (1977) The failures of success. *Milbank Memorial Fund Quarterly, 55,* 3–24

Gurland, B., Golden, R.R., Teresi, J.A. and Challop, J. (1984) The SHORT-CARE: an efficient instrument for the assessment of depression, dementia and disability. *Journal of Gerentology, 39,* 166–9

Gurland, B.J. and Wilder, D.E. (1984) The CARE interview revisited: development of an efficient, systematic clinical assessment. *Journal of Gerontology, 39,* 129–37

Hachinski, V.C., Iliff, L.D., Phil, M., Zilhka, E., Du Boulay, G.H., McAllister, V.L., Marshall, J., Ross Russell, R.W. and Symon, L. (1975) Cerebral blood flow in dementia. *Archives of Neurology, 32,* 632–7

Hachinski, V.C., Lassen, N.A. and Marshall, J. (1974) Multi-infarct dementia: a cause of mental deterioration in the elderly. *Lancet, 2,* 207–10

Hagnell, O., Lanke, J., Rorsman, B., Öhman, R. and Öjesjö, L. (1983) Current trends in the incidence of senile and multi-infarct dementia. *Archives of Psychiatry and Neurological Sciences, 233,* 423–38

Hanley, I.G. and Lusty, K. (1984) Memory aids in reality orientation: a single-case study. *Behaviour Research and Therapy, 22,* 709–12

Harris, C.S. and Ivory, P.B.C.B. (1976) An outcome evaluation of reality orientation therapy with geriatric patients in a state mental hospital. *Gerontologist, 16*, 496–504

Hart, S., Smith, C.M. and Swash, M. (1986) Assessing intellectual deterioration. *British Journal of Clinical Psychology, 25*, 119–24

Hasegawa, K., Honima, A., Sato, H., Aoba, A., Imai, Y., Yamaguchi, N. and Itami, A. (1984) The prevalence study of age-related dementia in the community [in Japanese]. *Geriatric Psychiatry, 1*, 94–105

Henderson, A.S. (1983) The coming epidemic of dementia. *Australian and New Zealand Journal of Psychiatry, 17*, 117–27

Henderson, A.S., Duncan-Jones, P. and Finlay-Jones, R.A. (1983) The reliability of the Geriatric Mental State Examination. *Acta Psychiatrica Scandinavica, 67*, 281–9

Henderson, A.S. and Jorm, A.F. (1986) *The problem of dementia in Australia*, Australian Government Publishing Service, Canberra

Henderson, B. (1980) Architectural. In E. Marshall and D. Eaton (eds), *Forgetting but not forgotten: residential care of mentally frail elderly people*, Uniting Church, Melbourne

Heston, L.L. (1981) Genetic studies of dementia: with emphasis on Parkinson's disease and Alzheimer's neuropathology. In J.A. Mortimer and L.M. Schuman (eds), *The epidemiology of dementia*, Oxford University Press, New York

Heston, L.L. (1982) Alzheimer's dementia and Down's syndrome: genetic evidence suggesting an association. *Annals of the New York Academy of Sciences, 396*, 29–37

Heston, L.L. (1984) Down's syndrome and Alzheimer's dementia: defining an association. *Psychiatric Developments, 4*, 287–94

Heston, L.L. and White, J. (1978) Pedigrees of 30 families with Alzheimer disease: associations with defective organization of microfilaments and microtubules. *Behavior Genetics, 8(4)*, 315–31

Heyman, A., Wilkinson, W.E., Hurwitz, B.J., Schmechel, D., Sigmon, A.H., Weinberg, T., Helms, M.J. and Swift, M. (1983) Alzheimer's disease: genetic aspects and associated clinical disorders. *Annals of Neurology, 14*, 507–15

Heyman, A., Wilkinson, W.E., Stafford, J.A., Helms, M.J., Sigmon, A.H. and Weinberg, T. (1984) Alzheimer's disease: a study of epidemiological aspects. *Annals of Neurology, 15(4)*, 335–41

Hier, D.B., Hagenlocker, K. and Shindler, A.G. (1985) Language disintegration in dementia: effects of etiology and severity. *Brain and Language, 25*, 117–33

Holzer, C.E., Tischler, G.L., Leaf, P.J. and Myers, J.K. (1984) An epidemiologic assessment of cognitive impairment in a community population. In *Research in Community and Mental Health*, Vol. 4, JAI Press, Greenwich, Connecticut

Hughes, C.P., Berg, L., Danziger, W.L., Coben, L.A. and Martin, R.L. (1982) A new clinical scale for the staging of dementia. *British Journal of Psychiatry, 140*, 566–72

Hunter, R., Dayan, A.D. and Wilson, J. (1972) Alzheimer's disease in one monozygotic twin. *Journal of Neurology, Neurosurgery and Psychiatry, 35*, 707–10

Hyman, B.T., Van Hoelsen, G.W., Damasio, A.R. and Barnes, C.L.

(1984) Alzheimer's disease: cell-specific pathology isolates the hippo-campal formation. *Science, 225,* 1168–70

Inglis, J. (1958) Psychological investigations of cognitive deficit in elderly psychiatric patients. *Psychological Bulletin, 55,* 197–214

Ivison, D.J. (1977) The Wechsler Memory Scale: preliminary findings towards an Australian standardisation. *Australian Psychologist, 12,* 303–12

Jenkins, J., Felce, D., Lunt, B. and Powell, L. (1977) Increasing engage-ment in activity of residents in old people's homes by providing recrea-tional materials. *Behaviour Research and Therapy, 15,* 429–34

Jorm, A.F. (1985) Subtypes of Alzheimer's dementia: a conceptual analysis and critical review. *Psychological Medicine, 15,* 543–53

Jorm, A.F. (1986a) Controlled and automatic information processing in senile dementia: a review. *Psychological Medicine, 16,* 77–88

Jorm, A.F. (1986b) Cognitive deficit in the depressed elderly: a review of some basic unresolved issues. *Australian and New Zealand Journal of Psychiatry, 20,* 11–22

Jorm, A.F. (1986c) Effects of cholinergic enhancement therapies on memory function in Alzheimer's disease: a meta-analysis of the literature. *Australian and New Zealand Journal of Psychiatry, 20,* 237–40

Kagan, A., Popper, J., Rhoads, G.G., Takeya, Y., Kato, H., Goode, G.B. and Marmot, M. (1976) Epidemiologic studies of coronary heart disease and stroke in Japanese men living in Japan, Hawaii, and California: prevalence of stroke. In P. Scheinberg (ed.), *Cerebrovascular diseases,* Raven Press, New York

Kahan, J., Kemp, B., Staples, F.R. and Brummel-Smith, K. (1985) Decreas-ing the burden in families caring for a relative with a dementing illness: a controlled study. *Journal of the American Geriatrics Society, 33,* 664–70

Kahn, R.L., Zarit, S.H., Hilbert, N.M. and Niederehe, G. (1975) Memory complaint and impairment in the aged: the effect of depression and altered brain function. *Archives of General Psychiatry, 32,* 1569–73

Karasawa, A., Kawashima, K. and Kasahara, H. (1982) Epidemiological study of the senile in Tokyo metropolitan area. *Proceedings of the World Psychiatric Association Regional Symposium,* 285–9

Katz, S., Ford, A.B., Moskowitz, R.W., Jackson, B.A. and Jaffe, M.W. (1963) Studies of illness in the aged. The Index of ADL: a standardized measure of biological and psychosocial function. *Journal of the American Medical Association, 185,* 914–19

Kay, D.W.K., Bergmann, K., Foster, E.M., McKechnie, A.A. and Roth, M. (1970) Mental illness and hospital usage in the elderly: a random sample followed up. *Comprehensive Psychiatry, 11,* 26–35

Kay, D.W.K., Henderson, A.S., Scott, R., Wilson, J., Rickwood, D. and Grayson, D.A. (1985) Dementia and depression among the elderly living in the Hobart community: the effect of the diagnostic criteria on the prevalence rates. *Psychological Medicine, 15,* 771–88

Kendrick, D.C., Gibson, A.J. and Moyes, I.C.A. (1979) The Revised Kendrick Battery: clinical studies, *British Journal of Social and Clinical Psychology, 18,* 329–40

Kiloh, L.G. (1961) Pseudo-dementia. *Acta Psychiatrica Scandinavica, 37,* 336–51

Kirshner, H.S., Webb, W.G. and Kelly, M.P. (1934) The naming disorder of dementia. *Neuropsychologica, 22,* 23–30

Kopelman, M.D. (1985) Multiple memory deficits in Alzheimer-type dementia: implications for pharmacotherapy. *Psychological Medicine, 15,* 527–41

Kraemer, H.C., Peabody, C.A., Tinklenberg, J.R. and Yesavage, J.A. (1983) Mathematical and empirical development of a test of memory for clinical and research use. *Psychological Bulletin, 94,* 367–80

Kuriansky, J. and Gurland, B. (1976) The Performance Test of Activities of Daily Living. *International Journal of Aging and Human Development, 7,* 343–52

Ladurner, G., Iliff, L.D. and Lechner, H. (1982) Clinical factors associated with dementia in ischaemic stroke. *Journal of Neurology, Neurosurgery and Psychiatry, 45,* 97–101

Langer, E.J. and Rodin, J. (1976) The effects of choice and enhanced personal responsibility for the aged: a field experiment in an institutional setting. *Journal of Personality and Social Psychology, 34,* 191–8

Langston, J.W. (1985) MPTP and Parkinson's disease. *Trends in Neurosciences, February,* 79–83

Lipowski, Z.J. (1983) Transient cognitive disorders (delirium, acute confusional states) in the elderly. *American Journal of Psychiatry, 140,* 1426–36

Liston, E.H. and LaRue, A. (1983) Clinical differentiation of primary degenerative and multi-infarct dementia: a critical review of the evidence. Part II: Pathological studies. *Biological Psychiatry, 18,* 1467–84

Little, A., Levy, R., Chuaqui-Kidd, P. and Hand, D. (1985) A double-blind, placebo controlled trial of high-dose lecithin in Alzheimer's disease. *Journal of Neurology, Neurosurgery and Psychiatry, 48,* 736–42

Mace, N.L. and Rabins, P.V. (1981) *The 36-hour day,* Johns Hopkins University Press, Baltimore

Mace, N.L., Rabins, P.V., Castleton, B., Cloke, C. and McEwan, E. (1985) *The 36-hour day,* Hodder and Stoughton, Sevenoaks, Kent

McGeer, P.L. (1986) Brain imaging in Alzheimer's disease. *British Medical Bulletin, 42,* 24–8

McHugh, P.R. and Folstein, M.F. (1979) Psychopathology of dementia: implications for neuropathology. In R. Katzman (ed.), *Congenital and acquired cognitive disorders,* Raven Press, New York

McPherson, F.M., Gamsu, C.V., Kiemle, G., Ritchie, S.M., Stanley, A.M. and Tregaskis, D. (1985) The concurrent validity of the survey version of the Clifton Assessment Procedures for the Elderly (CAPE). *British Journal of Clinical Psychology, 24,* 83–91

Margo, J.L., Robinson, J.R. and Corea, S. (1980) Referrals to a psychiatric service from old people's homes. *British Journal of Psychiatry, 136,* 396–401

Marsden, C.D. and Harrison, M.J.G. (1972) Outcome of investigation of patients with presenile dementia. *British Medical Journal, 2,* 249–52

Marshall, E. and Eaton, D. (1980) *Forgetting but not forgotten: residential care of mentally frail elderly people,* Uniting Church, Melbourne

Martin, A. and Fedio, P. (1983) Word production and comprehension in

Alzheimer's disease: the breakdown of semantic knowledge. *Brain and Language, 19,* 124–41

Matsuyama, H. (1983) Incidence of neurofibrillary change, senile plaques, and granulovacuolar, degeneration in aged individuals. In B. Reisberg (ed.), *Alzheimer's disease: the standard reference,* The Free Press, New York

Meacher, M. (1972) *Taken for a ride. Special residential homes for confused old people: a study of separatism in social policy,* Longman, London

Millar, H.R. (1981) Psychiatric morbidity in elderly surgical patients. *British Journal of Psychiatry, 138,* 17–20

Miller, D.F., Hicks, S.P., D'Amato, C.J. and Landis, J.R. (1984) A descriptive study of neuritic plaques and neurofibrillary tangles in an autopsy population. *American Journal of Epidemiology, 120,* 331–41

Miller, E. (1975) Impaired recall and the memory disturbance in presenile dementia. *British Journal of Social and Clinical Psychology, 14,* 73–9

Miller, E. (1977) The management of dementia: a review of some possibilities. *British Journal of Social and Clinical Psychology, 16,* 77–83

Miller, E. (1984) Verbal fluency as a function of a measure of verbal intelligence and in relation to different types of cerebral pathology. *British Journal of Clinical Psychology, 23,* 53–7

Miller, G.J. and Miller, N.E. (1975) Plasma-high-density-lipoprotein concentration and development of ischaemic heart-disease. *Lancet, 1,* 16–19

Miller, W.R. (1975) Psychological deficit in depression. *Psychological Bulletin, 82,* 238–60

Milner, P.M. (1966) *Physiological psychology,* Holt, Rinehart and Winston, New York

Mishara, B. (1978) Geriatric patients who improve in token economy and general milieu treatment programs: a multivariate analysis. *Journal of Consulting and Clinical Psychology, 46,* 1340–8

Moore, V. and Wyke, M.A. (1984) Drawing disability in patients with senile dementia. *Psychological Medicine, 14,* 97–105

Morris, R., Wheatley, J. and Britton, P. (1983) Retrieval from long-term memory in senile dementia; cued recall revisited. *British Journal of Clinical Psychology, 22,* 141–2

Morrison, J.H., Rogers, J., Scherr, S., Benoit, R. and Bloom, F.E. (1985) Somatostatin immunoreactivity in neurotic plaques of Alzheimer patients. *Nature, 314,* 90–4

Mortimer, J.A., French, L.R. Hutton, J.T. and Schuman, L.M. (1985) Head injury as a risk factor for Alzheimer's disease. *Neurology, 35,* 264–7

Moscovitch, M. (1982) A neuropsychological approach to perception and memory in normal and pathological aging. In F.I.M. Craik and S. Trehub (eds), *Aging and cognitive processes,* Plenum Press, New York

Muckle, T.J. and Roy, J.R. (1985) High-density lipoprotein cholesterol in differential diagnosis of senile dementia. *Lancet, 1,* 1191–3

Murphy, E. (1982) Social origins of depression in old age. *British Journal of Psychiatry, 141,* 135–42

Nebes, R.D., Martin, D.C. and Horn, L.C. (1984) Sparing of semantic memory in Alzheimer's disease. *Journal of Abnormal Psychology, 93,* 321–30

Nelson, H.E. and McKenna, P. (1975) The use of current reading ability in the assessment of dementia. *British Journal of Social and Clinical Psychology, 14,* 259–67

Nelson, H.E. and O'Connell, A. (1978) Dementia: the estimation of premorbid intelligence levels using the New Adult Reading Test. *Cortex, 14,* 234–44

Newton, E. (1979) *This bed my centre,* Virago, London

Ogden, M., Kellett, J.M., Merryfield, P. and Millard, P.H. (1984) Practical aspects of automated testing of the elderly. *Bulletin of the British Psychological Society, 37,* 148–9

Parsons, P.L. (1965) Mental health of Swansea's old folk. *British Journal of Preventive and Social Medicine, 19,* 43–7

Pattie, A.H. (1981) A survey version of the Clifton Assessment Procedures for the Elderly (CAPE). *British Journal of Clinical Psychology, 20,* 173–8

Pattie, A.H. and Gilleard, C.J. (1975) A brief psychogeriatric assessment schedule: validation against psychiatric diagnosis and discharge from hospital. *British Journal of Psychiatry, 127,* 489–93

Pattie, A.H. and Gilleard, C.J. (1979) *Manual of the Clifton Assessment Procedures for the Elderly (CAPE),* Hodder and Stoughton, Sevenoaks, Kent

Pearce, F. (1985) Acid rain may cause senile dementia. *New Scientist, 25 April,* 7

Pérez, E.L. and Silverman, M. (1984) Delirium: the often overlooked diagnosis. *International Journal of Psychiatry in Medicine, 14,* 181–9

Perl, D.P. and Brody, A.R. (1980) Alzheimer's disease: X-ray spectrometric evidence of aluminium accumulation in neurofibrillary tangle-bearing neurons. *Science, 208,* 297–9

Perry, E.K., Tomlinson, B.E., Blessed, G., Bergmann, K., Gibson, P.H. and Perry, R.H. (1978) Correlation of cholinergic abnormalities with senile plaques and mental test scores in senile dementia. *British Medical Journal, 2,* 1457–9

Pinessi, L., Rainero, I., Angelini, G., Asteggiano, G., Bianco, C., Festa, T., Giachino, R. and Bergamasco, B. (1983) I fattori di rischio nelle sindromi demenziali primarie. *Minerva Psichiatrica, 24,* 87–91

Plum, F. (1979) Dementia: an approaching epidemic. *Nature, 279,* 372–3

Powell-Proctor, L. and Miller, E. (1982) Reality orientation: a critical appraisal. *British Journal of Psychiatry, 140,* 457–63

Prineas, R.J. (1971) Cerebrovascular disease occurrence in Australia. *Medical Journal of Australia, 2,* 509–15

Prusiner, S.B. (1982) Novel proteinaceous infectious particles cause scrapie. *Science, 216,* 136–44

Prusiner, S.B. (1984) Some speculations about prions, amyloid and Alzheimer's disease. *New England Journal of Medicine, 310,* 661–3

Rabins, P.V. and Folstein, M.F. (1982) Delirium and dementia: diagnostic criteria and fatality rates. *British Journal of Psychiatry, 140,* 149–53

Rabins, P.V., Merchant, A. and Nestadt, G. (1984) Criteria for diagnosing reversible dementia caused by depression — validation by 2 year follow-up.

British Journal of Psychiatry, 144, 488–92

Reifler, B.V., Larson, E. and Hanley, R. (1982) Co-existence of cognitive impairment and depression in geriatric outpatients. *American Journal of Psychiatry, 139,* 623–6

Reisberg, B. (1981) Empirical studies in senile dementia with metabolic enhancers and agents that alter blood flow and oxygen utilization. In T. Crook and S. Gershon (eds), *Strategies for the development of an effective treatment for senile dementia,* Mark Powley Associates, New Canaan, Conn.

Roberts, G.W., Crow, T.J. and Polak, J.M. (1985) Location of neuronal tangles in somatostatin neurones in Alzheimer's disease. *Nature, 314,* 92–4

Rodin, J. and Langer, E.J. (1977) Long-term effects of a control-relevant intervention with the institutionalized aged. *Journal of Personality and Social Psychology, 35,* 897–902

Rossor, M.N., Iversen, L.L., Reynolds, G.P. Mountjoy, C.Q. and Roth, M. (1984) Early and late onset types of Alzheimer's disease. *British Medical Journal, 288,* 961–4

Roth, M., Tym, E., Mountjoy, C.Q., Huppert, F.A., Hendrie, H., Verma, S. and Goddard, R. (1986) CAMDEX: A standardized instrument for the diagnosis of mental disorder in the elderly with special reference to the early detection of dementia. *British Journal of Psychiatry, 149,* 698–709

Royal College of Physicians of London, Committee on Geriatrics. (1981) Organic mental impairment in the elderly. Implications for research, education and the provision of services. *Journal of the Royal College of Physicians of London, 15,* 141–67

Ruddell, H.V. and Bradshaw, C.M. (1982) On the estimation of premorbid intellectual functioning: validation of Nelson and McKenna's formula, and some new normative data. *British Journal of Clinical Psychology, 21,* 159–65

Schonell, F.J. and Schonnell, F.E. (1952) *Diagnostic and Attainment Testing,* Oliver and Boyd, Edinburgh

Seltzer, B. and Sherwin, I. (1986) Fingerprint pattern differences in early- and late-onset primary degenerative dementia. *Archives of Neurology, 43,* 665–8

Serby, M., Corwin, J., Jordan, B., Novatt, A. and Rotrosen, J. (1984) Side effects of scopolamine administration. *American Journal of Psychiatry, 141,* 1010

Shore, D. and Wyatt, R.J. (1983) Aluminium and Alzheimer's disease. *Journal of Nervous and Mental Disease, 171,* 553–8

Siegel, J.S. and Hoover, S.L. (1982) Demographic aspects of the health of the elderly to the year 2000 and beyond. *World Health Statistics Quarterly, 35,* 133–202

Slater, E. and Cowie, V. (1971) *The genetics of mental health disorders,* Oxford University Press, London

Smith, J.S. and Kiloh, L.G. (1981) The investigation of dementia: results in 200 consecutive admissions. *Lancet, 1,* 824–7

Struble, R.G., Cork, L.C., Whitehouse, P.J. and Price, D.L. (1982) Cholinergic innervation in neuritic plaques. *Science, 216,* 413–15

Sulkava, R., Haltia, M., Paetau, A., Wikström, J. and Palo, J. (1983) Accuracy of clinical diagnosis in primary degenerative dementia: correlation with neuropathological findings. *Journal of Neurology, Neurosurgery and Psychiatry, 46,* 9–13

Ueda, K., Omae, T., Hirota, Y., Takeshita, M., Katsuki, S., Tanaka, K. and Enjoji, M. (1981) Decreasing trend in incidence and mortality from stroke in Hisayama residents, Japan. *Stroke, 12,* 154–60

Ulrich, J. (1985) Alzheimer changes in nondemented patients younger than sixty-five: possible early stages of Alzheimer's disease and senile dementia of Alzheimer type. *Annals of Neurology, 17,* 273–7

Wechsler, D. and Stone, C.P. (1945) *Wechsler Memory Scale,* The Psychological Corporation, New York

Weingartner, H., Grafman, J., Boutelle, W., Kaye, W. and Martin, P.R. (1983) Forms of memory failure. *Science, 221,* 380–2

Weingartner, H., Kaye, W., Smallberg, S.A., Ebert, M.H., Gillin, J.C. and Sitaram, N. (1981) Memory failures in progressive idiopathic dementia. *Journal of Abnormal Psychology, 90,* 187–96

Weinreb, H.J. (1985) Fingerprint patterns in Alzheimer's disease. *Archives of Neurology, 42,* 50–4

Wells, C.E. (1979) Pseudodementia. *American Journal of Psychiatry, 136,* 895–900

Weyerer, S. (1983) Mental disorders among the elderly: true prevalence and use of medical services. *Archives of Gerontology and Geriatrics, 2,* 11–12

Whalley, L.J., Carothers, A.D., Collyer, S., de Mey, R. and Frackiewicz, A. (1982) A study of familial factors in Alzheimer's disease. *British Journal of Psychiatry, 140,* 249–56

Whalley, L.J. and Holloway, S. (1985) Non-random geographical distribution of Alzheimer's presenile dementia in Edinburgh, 1953–76. *Lancet, 1,* 578

Wilkins, R.H. and Brody, M.D. (1969) Alzheimer's disease. *Archives of Neurology, 21,* 109

Williamson, J., Stokoe, I.H., Gray, M.S., Fisher, M., Smith, A., McGhee, A. and Stephenson, E. (1964) Old people at home: their unreported needs. *Lancet. 1,* 1117–20

Wilson, R.S., Rosenbaum, G. and Brown, G. (1979) The problem of premorbid intelligence in neuropsychological assessment. *Journal of Clinical Neuropsychology, 1,* 49–53

Wischik, C.M., Crowther, R.A., Stewart, M. and Roth, M. (1985) Subunit structure of paired helical filaments in Alzheimer's disease. *Journal of Cell Biology, 100,* 1905–12

Wisniewski, H.M. (1983) Neuritic (senile) and amyloid plaques. In B. Reisberg (ed.), *Alzheimer's disease: The standard reference,* The Free Press, New York

Wisniewski, K.E. Wisniewski, H.M. and Wen, G.Y. (1985) Occurrence of neuropathological changes and dementia of Alzheimer's disease in Down's syndrome. *Annals of Neurology, 17,* 278–82

Wong, D.F., Wagner, H.N., Dannals, R.F. *et al.* (1984) Effects of age on dopamine and serotonin receptors measured by positron tomography in the living human brain. *Science, 226,* 1393–6

World Health Organization (1982) Special issue on public health implications of aging. *World Health Statistics Quarterly*, 35, No. 3/4

Wright, A.F. and Whalley, L.J. (1984) Genetics, ageing and dementia. *British Journal of Psychiatry*, 145, 20–38

Young, R.C., Manley, M.W. and Alexopoulos, G.S. (1985) 'I don't know' responses in elderly depressives and in dementia. *Journal of the American Geriatrics Society*, 33, 253–7

Zanetti, O., Rozzini, R., Bianchetti, A. and Trabucchi, M. (1985) HDL-cholesterol in dementia. *Lancet*, 2, 43

Zarit, S.H., Reever, K.E. and Bach-Peterson, J. (1980) Relatives of the impaired elderly: correlates of feelings of burden. *Gerontologist*, 20, 649–55

Author Index

Subject Index